EXERCISES FOR
ARTHRITIS

By Erin Rohan O'Driscoll R.N., M.A.

with a Foreword by
John D. Hubbell, MD
Photography by Peter Field Peck

Healthy Living Books

New York

A Healthy Living Book
Hatherleigh Press
5–22 46th Avenue, Suite 200
Long Island City, NY 11101
www.healthylivingbooks.com

Library of Congress Cataloging-in-Publication data available upon request.
ISBN: 1-57826-166-X

Names of medications are typically followed by ® symbols, but these symbols are not stated in this book.

Brand names included in this book are provided as examples only, and their inclusion does not imply an endorsement. Also, if a particular brand name is not mentioned, this does not mean or imply that the product is unsatisfactory

All forms of exercise pose some inherent risks. The information in this book is meant to supplement, not replace, proper exercise training. Before practicing the exercises in this book, be sure that your equipment is well maintained. Do not take risks beyond your level of experience, training, and fitness. The exercise and dietary programs in this book are not intended as a substitute for any exercise routine or treatment or dietary regimen that may have been prescribed by your doctor. As with all exercise and dietary programs, you should get your doctor's approval before beginning. The author(s), editors, and publisher advice readers to take full responsibility for their safety and know their limits.

Healthy Living Books titles are available for bulk purchase, special promotions, and premiums. For information about reselling and special purchase opportunities, please call 1-800-528-2550 and ask for the Special Sales Manager.

Cover and Interior Design by Deborah Miller

10 9 8 7 6 5 4 3 2 1
Printed in Canada

I dedicate this book to the memory of
my maternal grandmother, Katherine Woreth,
who suffered with rheumatoid arthritis and osteoarthritis.

Acknowledgements

Special thanks to the National Institute of Arthritis and Musculoskeletal and Skin Diseases for the information in Part I. Much of the material has been reprinted from its publications *Handout on Health: Osteoarthritis; Handout on Health: Rheumatoid Arthritis;* and *Questions and Answers about Fibromyalgia.*

Table of Contents

Foreword

As an Orthopaedist I treat patients with arthritic problems on a daily basis. In the United States, estimates of arthritis range from as low as 6 percent of the adult population to as high as 90 percent of adults over 40 years of age. In a 2000 report from the National Center for Health Statistics, 32.9 million Americans (about 23 percent of the adult population) reported that their physicians told them that they have some type of arthritis. Increased life expectancy coupled with a more active older population has led to a greater prevalence of symptomatic arthritis. The weight bearing joints, especially the knees and hips, are most susceptible to the development of arthritic conditions. In the past, patients suffering from arthritic pain were given the option to live with the pain or be limited to life in a wheelchair. Thankfully, these options are rarely entertained in today's treatment protocols.

The main goal of my treatment is to restore a patient's quality of life using programs to control abuse and pain while maintaining motion and strength. The slogan of the 80's, "no pain no gain" does not have a place in the treatment plan and often makes symptoms worse. Furthermore, rest alone is not an acceptable option. Rest leads to muscular weakness, which can further weaken the extremity and place greater demands on an ailing joint creating a vicious cycle. Modification of activities is often the solution. Supervised Physical Therapy, Yoga, and Pilates can be very useful in maintaining the strength and motion of the arthritic joint. The use of medications and supplements are also useful in certain cases. In the most advanced stages, when non-operative treatment options fail, surgery can help to restore a patients' quality of life.

The great value of this book is that it clearly outlines the history, symptoms and progression of different arthritic conditions. The various treatment options are discussed in a user friendly manner. The exercises, which are crucial to maintaining strength and function, are described in great detail and easy to perform without any costly equipment. Finally, organized exercise and strengthening programs are discussed concisely and provide a gradual pace for arthritis sufferers to follow. The information contained in this book can provide invaluable information allowing patients to become more involved with their success while facing arthritic pain.

—*John D. Hubbell, MD*
March 2004

Author's Note

When you have arthritis, your most important concerns are managing your symptoms, maintaining your independence, and enjoying life. This book will help you live your life to the fullest despite arthritis. You can accomplish this by following a program of exercise designed specifically for your arthritic condition.

According to the American College of Sports Medicine, regular physical activity is necessary for maintaining normal muscular strength and joint structure and function.

When performed in the range recommended for health, physical activity is not associated with joint damage or the development of osteoarthritis. In fact, it may be beneficial for many people with arthritis.*

Regular exercise can increase your energy level and decrease arthritis-related limitations when you perform physical tasks. Your exercise program should be tailored to your own physical condition, type, and severity of your arthritis and your flexibility and strength. Pay attention to your body sensations and adjust your exercise selection, intensity, and frequency accordingly.

*American College of Sports Medicine, *Certified News*, December 1996.

Part I: Introduction

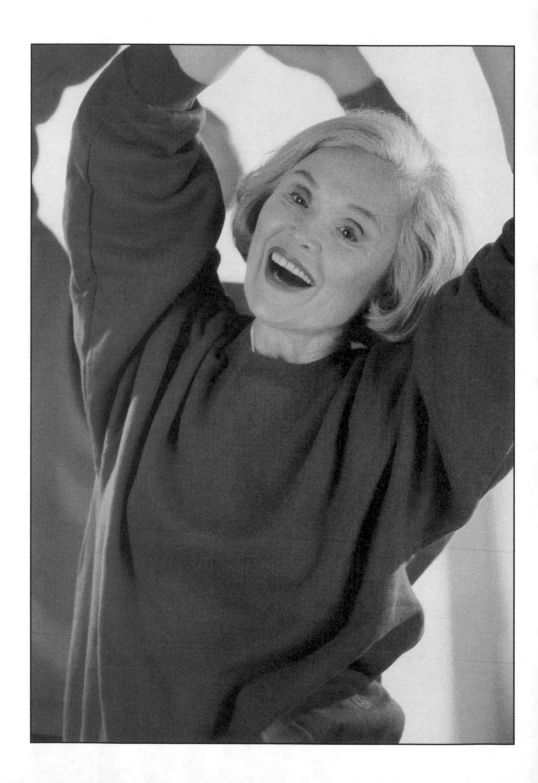

1

Arthritis Basics

There are over 100 forms of arthritis and other rheumatic diseases. These diseases may cause pain, stiffness, and swelling in joints and other supporting structures of the body such as muscles, tendons, ligaments, and bones. Some forms can also affect other parts of the body, including various internal organs.

Many people use the word "arthritis" to refer to all rheumatic diseases. However, the word literally means joint inflammation; that is, swelling, redness, heat, and pain caused by tissue injury or disease in the joint. The many different kinds of arthritis comprise just a portion of the rheumatic diseases. Some rheumatic diseases are described as connective tissue diseases because they affect the body's connective tissue—the supporting framework of the body and its internal organs. Others are known as autoimmune diseases because they are caused by a problem in which the immune system harms the body's own healthy tissues. Examples of some rheumatic diseases are:

+ Ankylosing spondylitis
+ Fibromyalgia
+ Gout
+ Juvenile rheumatoid arthritis
+ Osteoarthritis
+ Rheumatoid arthritis
+ Scleroderma
+ Systemic lupus erythematosus

In this book, we focus specifically on three types of arthritis: osteoarthritis, rheumatoid arthritis, and fibromyalgia.

Sixteen million people nationally have osteoarthritis. It affects men more frequently up to age 45 years; after age 55, it is more common in women. In comparison, 2.5 million people have rheumatoid arthritis (1 percent of the U.S. population) with women outnumbering men 3 to 1. The annual medical care cost for the treatment of rheumatoid arthritis is $4,798 for each single person affected.

A surprising fact is that fibromyalgia is more common than rheumatoid arthritis. It affects approximately 2 percent of the general population.

Population affected with Arthritis

Osteoarthritis	20.7 million
Fibromyalgia	3.7 million
Rheumatoid	2.1 million
Juvenile arthritis	285, 000

Sources: *American Journal of Nursing*, Nov. 2000; *The Arthritis Foundation*

2

Osteoarthritis

O steoarthritis is the most common type of arthritis, especially among older people. Sometimes it is called degenerative joint disease or osteoarthrosis.

Osteoarthritis is a joint disease that mostly affects the cartilage. Cartilage is the slippery tissue that covers the ends of bones in a joint. Healthy cartilage allows bones to glide over one another. It also absorbs energy from the shock of physical movement. In osteoarthritis, the surface layer of cartilage breaks down and wears away. This allows bones under the cartilage to rub together, causing pain, swelling, and loss of motion of the joint. Over time, the joint may lose its normal shape. Also, bone spurs—small growths called osteophytes—may grow on the edges of the joint. Bits of bone or cartilage can break off and float inside the joint space. This causes more pain and damage.

People with osteoarthritis usually have joint pain and limited movement. Unlike some other forms of arthritis, osteoarthritis affects only joints and not internal organs. For example, rheumatoid arthritis—the second most common form of arthritis—affects other parts of the body besides the joints. It begins at a younger age than osteoarthritis, causes swelling and redness in joints, and may make people feel sick, tired, and (uncommonly) feverish.

Who Has Osteoarthritis?

Osteoarthritis is one of the most frequent causes of physical disability among adults. More than 20 million people in the United States have the disease. By 2030, 20 percent of Americans—about 70 million people—will have passed their 65th birthday and will be at risk for osteoarthritis. Some younger people get osteoarthritis from joint injuries, but osteoarthritis most often occurs in older people. In fact, more than half of the population age 65 or older would show x-ray evidence of osteoarthritis in at least one joint. Both men and women have the disease. Before age 45, more men than women have osteoarthritis, whereas after age 45, it is more common in women.

How Does Osteoarthritis Affect People?

Osteoarthritis affects each person differently. In some people, it progresses quickly; in others, the symptoms are more serious. Scientists do not know yet what causes the disease, but they suspect a combination of factors, including being overweight, the aging process, joint injury, and stresses on the joints from certain jobs and sports activities.

What Areas Does Osteoarthritis Affect?

Osteoarthritis most often occurs at the ends of the fingers, thumbs, neck, lower back, knees, and hips.

Osteoarthritis hurts people in more than their joints: Their finances and lifestyles also are affected.

Financial effects include the cost of treatment and wages lost because of disability. Lifestyle effects include anxiety, depression, feelings of helplessness, job limitations, limitations on daily activities, and trouble participating in everyday personal and family joys and responsibilities.

Despite these challenges, most people with osteoarthritis can lead active and productive lives. They succeed by using osteoarthritis treatment strategies, such as the following:

+ Learning self-care and having a "good-health attitude."

+ Pain relief medications

+ Patient education and support programs

+ Rest and exercise

Osteoarthritis Basics: The Joint and Its Parts

Most joints—the place where two moving bones come together—are designed to allow smooth movement between the bones and to absorb shock from movements like walking or repetitive movements. The joint is made up of:

Cartilage. A dense but slippery coating on the end of each bone. Cartilage, which breaks down and wears away in osteoarthritis, is described in more detail below.

Joint capsule. A tough membrane sac that holds all the bones and other joint parts together.

Synovium. A thin membrane inside the joint capsule.

Synovial fluid. A fluid that lubricates the joint and keeps the cartilage smooth and healthy.

Ligaments, tendons, and muscles. Tissues that keep the bones stable and allow the joint to bend and move. Ligaments are tough, cord-like tissues that connect one bone to another. Tendons are tough, fibrous cords that connect muscles to bones. Muscles are bundles of specialized cells that contract to produce movement when stimulated by nerves.

How Do You Know if You Have Osteoarthritis?

Usually, osteoarthritis comes on slowly. Early in the disease, joints may ache after physical work or exercise. Osteoarthritis can occur in any joint. Most often it occurs at the hands, knees, hips, or spine.

Hands. Osteoarthritis of the fingers is one type of osteoarthritis that seems to have some hereditary characteristics; that is, it runs in families. More women than men have it, and they develop it especially after menopause. In osteoarthritis, small, bony knobs appear on the end joints of the fingers. They are called *Heberden's nodes.* Similar knobs, called *Bouchard's nodes,* can appear on the middle joints of

A Healthy Joint

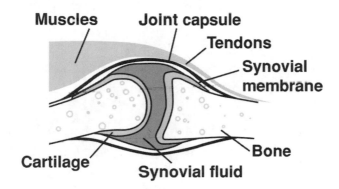

A Joint with Osteoarthritis

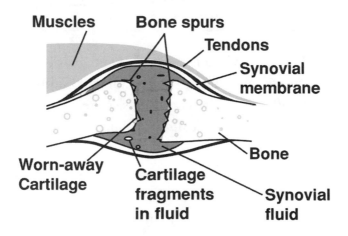

Cartilage: The Key to Healthy Joints

Cartilage is 65 to 80 percent water. Three other components make up the rest of cartilage tissue. collagen, proteoglycans, and chondrocytes.

Collagen. A fibrous protein. Collagen is also the building block of skin, tendon, bone, and other connective tissues.

Proteoglycans. A combination of proteins and sugars. Strands of proteoglycans and collagen weave together and form a mesh-like tissue. This allows cartilage to flex and absorb physical shock.

Chondrocytes. Cells that are found all through the cartilage. They mainly help cartilage stay healthy and grow. Sometimes, however, they release substances called enzymes that destroy collagen and other proteins. Researchers are trying to learn more about chondrocytes.

the fingers. Fingers can become enlarged and gnarled, and they may ache or be stiff and numb. The base of the thumb joint also is commonly affected by osteoarthritis. Osteoarthritis of the hands can be helped by medications, splints, or heat treatment.

Knees. The knees are the body's primary weight-bearing joints. For this reason, they are among the joints most commonly affected by osteoarthritis. They may be stiff, swollen, and painful, making it hard to walk, climb, and get in and out of chairs and bathtubs. If not treated, osteoarthritis in the knees can lead to disability. Medications, weight-loss, exercise, and walking aids can reduce pain and disability. In severe cases, knee replacement surgery may be helpful.

Hips. Osteoarthritis in the hip can cause pain, stiffness, and severe disability. People may feel the pain in their hips, or in their groin, inner thigh, buttocks, or knees. Walking aids, such as canes or walkers, can reduce stress on the hip. Osteoarthritis in the hip may limit moving and bending. This can make daily activities such as dressing and foot care a challenge. Walking aids, medication, and exercise can help relieve pain and improve motion. The doctor may recommend hip replacement if the pain is severe and not relieved by other methods.

Spine. Stiffness and pain in the neck or in the lower back can result from osteoarthritis of the spine. Weakness or numbness of the arms or legs also can result. Some people feel better when they sleep on a firm mattress or sit using back-support pillows. Others find it helps to use heat treatments or to follow an exercise program that strengthens the back and abdominal muscles. In severe cases, the doctor may suggest surgery to reduce pain and help restore function.

The Warning Signs of Osteoarthritis

+ Steady or intermittent pain in a joint

+ Stiffness in a joint after getting out of bed or sitting for a long time

+ Swelling or tenderness in one or more joints

+ A crunching feeling or the sound of bone rubbing on bone

+ Hot, red, or tender? Probably not osteoarthritis. Check with your doctor about other causes, such as rheumatoid arthritis.

+ Pain? Not always. In fact, only a third of people whose X rays show evidence of osteoarthritis report pain or other symptoms.

How Do Doctors Diagnose Osteoarthritis?

No single test can diagnose osteoarthritis. Most doctors use a combination of the following methods to diagnose the disease and rule out other conditions.

Treatment Approaches to Osteoarthritis

+ Exercise
+ Weight control
+ Rest and joint care
+ Pain relief techniques

+ Medicines
+ Alternative therapies
+ Surgery

Clinical history. The doctor begins by asking the patient to describe the symptoms, and when and how the condition started. Good doctor-patient communication is important. The doctor can give a better assessment if the patient gives a good description of pain, stiffness, and joint function, and how they have changed over time. It also is important for the doctor to know how the condition affects the patient's work and daily life. Finally, the doctor also needs to know about other medical conditions and whether the patient is taking any medicines.

Physical examination. The doctor will check the patient's general health, including checking reflexes and muscle strength. Joints bothering the patient will be examined. The doctor will also observe the patient's ability to walk, bend, and carry out activities of daily living.

X rays. Doctors X ray to see how much joint damage has been done. X rays of the affected joint can show such things as cartilage loss, bone damage, and bone spurs. But there often is a big difference between the severity of osteoarthritis as shown by the X ray and the degree of pain and disability felt by the patient. Also, X rays may not show early osteoarthritis damage, before much cartilage loss has taken place.

Other tests. The doctor may order blood tests to rule out other causes of symptoms. Another common test is called joint aspiration, which involves drawing fluid from the joint for examination.

It usually is not difficult to tell whether a patient has osteoarthritis. It is more difficult to tell whether the disease is causing the patient's symptoms. Osteoarthritis is so common—especially in older people—that symptoms seemingly caused by the disease actually may be due to other medical conditions. The doctor will try to find out what is causing the symptoms by ruling out other disorders and identifying conditions that may make the symptoms worse. The severity of symptoms in osteoarthritis is influenced greatly by the patient's attitude, anxiety, depression, and daily activity level.

How Is Osteoarthritis Treated?

Most successful treatment programs involve a combination of treatments tailored to the patient's needs, lifestyle, and health. Osteoarthritis treatment has four general goals:

+ Improve joint care through rest and exercise.

+ Maintain an acceptable body weight.

+ Control pain with medicine and other measures.

+ Achieve a healthy lifestyle.

Osteoarthritis treatment plans often include ways to manage pain and improve function. Such plans can involve exercise, rest and joint care, pain relief, weight control, medicines, surgery, and non-traditional treatment approaches.

Exercise. Research shows that exercise is one of the best treatments for osteoarthritis. Exercise can improve mood and outlook, decrease pain, increase flexibility, improve the heart and blood flow, maintain weight, and promote general physical fitness. Exercise is also inexpensive and, if done correctly, has few negative side effects. The amount and form of exercise will depend on which joints are involved, how stable the joints are, and whether a joint replacement has already been done.

Rest and joint care. Treatment plans include regularly scheduled rest. Patients must learn to recognize the body's signals, and know when to stop or slow down, which prevents pain caused by overexertion. Some patients find that relaxation techniques, stress reduction, and biofeedback help. Some use canes and splints to protect joints and take pressure off them. Splints or braces provide extra support for weakened joints. They also keep the joint in proper position during sleep or activity. Splints should be used only for limited periods because joints and muscles need to be exercised to prevent stiffness and weakness. An occupational therapist or a doctor can help the patient get a properly fitting splint.

Nondrug pain relief. People with osteoarthritis may find nondrug ways to relieve pain. Warm towels, hot packs, or a warm bath or shower to apply moist heat to the joint can relieve pain and stiffness. In some cases, cold packs (a bag of ice or frozen vegetables wrapped in a towel can relieve pain or numb the sore area. (Check with a doctor or physical therapist to find out if heat or cold is the best treatment.) Water therapy in a heated pool or whirlpool also may relieve pain and stiff-

Tips for Weight Control

1. Make changes slowly. At each meal, think: How can I modify what I'm eating right now to make it more healthy? It may be eliminating butter or salt. Take a larger vegetable portion and less meat, or skip the bread with your meal.

2. Most people don't drink enough water. Do you? Some people say "I hate drinking water; it's so boring." Fill a water bottle with half juice and half water and keep it with you throughout the day. Take sips periodically. It keeps your appetite satisfied and you will be getting the water you need.

3. Exercise daily, even if it's only 15 or 20 minutes. Find a way to fit it into your daily routine. You will feel much better afterward.

4. Keep records of what you eat each day and the time—even the small bite of your grandson's pizza or the piece of candy you grabbed on your way out the door. Keep a daily exercise/activity log book. Write down anything that would be considered active; for example, if you walked the parking lot of the mall, instead of being dropped off at the door, write it down. Record it as 3-minute walk from car to store. Do you get the idea? In addition, record all the exercises you may have done that day. Compare your food list with your exercise/activity list. If the food list is a lot longer, then you have a problem. You are probably eating more calories than you are burning. Keeping a record will help you be more mindful about what you are eating, and help identify bad eating habits, such as eating right before you go to bed. It will motivate you to perform the exercises suggested in this book.

ness. For osteoarthritis in the knee, patients may wear insoles or cushioned shoes to redistribute weight and reduce joint stress.

Weight control. Osteoarthritis patients who are overweight or obese need to lose weight; obese women have four times the occurrence of osteoarthritis of the knee than women of average weight. Weight loss can reduce stress on weight-bearing joints and limit further injury. A dietitian can help patients develop healthy eating habits.

Medicines. Doctors prescribe medicines to eliminate or reduce pain and to improve functioning. Doctors consider a number of factors when choosing medicines for their patients with osteoarthritis. Two important factors are the intensity of the pain and the potential side effects of the medicine. Patients must use medicines carefully and tell their doctors about any changes that occur.

The following types of medicines are commonly used in treating osteoarthritis:

Acetaminophen is a pain reliever (for example, Tylenol) that does not reduce swelling. Acetaminophen does not irritate the stomach and is less likely than nonsteroidal anti-inflammatory drugs (NSAIDs) to cause long-term side effects. Research has shown that acetaminophen relieves pain as effectively as NSAIDs for many patients with osteoarthritis. *Warning:* People with liver disease, people who drink alcohol heavily, and those taking blood-thinning medicines or NSAIDs should use acetaminophen with caution.

NSAIDs (nonsteroidal anti-inflammatory drugs): Many NSAIDs are used to treat osteoarthritis. Patients can buy some over the counter (for example, aspirin, Advil, Motrin IB, Aleve, ketoprofen). Others require a prescription. All NSAIDs work similarly: they fight inflammation and relieve pain. However, each NSAID is a different chemical, and each has a slightly different effect on the body.

Side effects. NSAIDs can cause stomach irritation or, less often, they can affect kidney function. The longer a person uses NSAIDs, the more likely he or she is to have side effects, ranging from mild to serious. Many other drugs cannot be taken when a patient is being treated with NSAIDs because NSAIDs alter the way the body uses or eliminates these other drugs. Check with your health care provider or pharmacist before you take NSAIDs in addition to another medication. Also, NSAIDs sometimes are associated with serious gastrointestinal problems, including ulcers, bleeding, and perforation of the stomach or intestine. People over age 65 and those with any history of ulcers or gastrointestinal bleeding should use NSAIDs with caution.

COX-2 inhibitors. Several new NSAIDs—valdecoxib (Bextra), celecoxib (Celebrex), and rofecoxib (Vioxx)—from a class of drugs known as COX-2 inhibitors are now being used to treat osteoarthritis. These medicines reduce inflammation similarly to traditional NSAIDs, but they cause fewer gastrointestinal side effects. However, these medications occasionally are associated with harmful reactions ranging from mild to severe.

Other medications. Doctors may prescribe several other medicines for osteoarthritis, including the following:

Topical pain-relieving creams, rubs, and sprays (for example, capsaicin cream), which are applied directly to the skin.

Mild narcotic painkillers, which—although very effective—may be addictive and are not commonly used.

Corticosteroids, powerful anti-inflammatory hormones made naturally in the body or man-made for use as medicine. Corticosteroids may be injected into the affected joints to temporarily relieve pain. This is a short-term measure, generally not recommended for more than two or three treatments per year. Oral corticosteroids should not be used to treat osteoarthritis.

Hyaluronic acid, a medicine for joint injection, used to treat osteoarthritis of the knee. This substance is a normal component of the joint, involved in joint lubrication and nutrition.

Questions To Ask Your Doctor or Pharmacist About Medicines

+ How often should I take this medicine?

+ Should I take this medicine with food or between meals?

+ What side effects can I expect?

+ Should I take this medicine with the other prescription medicines I take?

+ Should I take this medicine with the over-the-counter medicines I take?

Most medicines used to treat osteoarthritis have side effects, so it is important for people to learn about the medicines they take. Even nonprescription drugs should be checked. Several groups of patients are at high risk for side effects from NSAIDs, such as people with a history of peptic ulcers or digestive tract bleeding, people taking oral corticosteroids or anticoagulants (blood thinners), smokers, and people who consume alcohol. Some patients may be able to help reduce side effects by taking some medicines with food. Others should avoid stomach irritants such as alcohol, tobacco, and caffeine. Some patients try to protect their stomachs by taking other medicines that coat the stomach or block stomach acids. These measures help, but they are not always completely effective.

Surgery. For many people, surgery helps relieve the pain and disability of osteoarthritis. Surgery may be performed to:

+ Remove loose pieces of bone and cartilage from the joint if they are causing mechanical symptoms of buckling or locking

+ Replace joints.

+ Reposition bones

+ Resurface (smooth out) bones

Surgeons may replace affected joints with artificial joints called prostheses. These joints can be made from metal alloys, high-density plastic, and ceramic material. They can be joined to bone surfaces by special cements. Artificial joints can last 10 to 15 years or longer. About 10 percent of artificial joints may need revision. Surgeons choose the design and components of prostheses according to their patient's weight, sex, age, activity level, and other medical conditions.

The decision to use surgery depends on several factors. Both the surgeon and the patient consider the patient's level of disability, the intensity of pain, the interference with the patient's lifestyle, the patient's age, and occupation. Currently, more than 80 percent of osteoarthritis surgery cases involve replacing the hip or knee joint. After surgery and rehabilitation, the patient usually feels less pain and swelling, and can move more easily.

Nontraditional approaches. Among the alternative therapies used to treat osteoarthritis are the following:

Glucosamine and Chondroitin

Many doctors are now recommending natural substances for the treatment of osteoarthritis. This may be in response to the public demand for a more holistic approach to the treatment of various diseases.

Glucosamine is a natural substance found in the body. It plays an important role in the health of your cartilage. It's made from the combination of glucose (sugar) and a protein. As you age, you lose some of the glucosamine in your cartilage. This can lead to the breakdown and thinning of cartilage.

Chondroitin, like glucosamine, is formed from a sugar-like molecule. It is found in cartilage tissue and help it withstand pressure for weight-bearing activities. Some studies have shown that chondroitin may interfere with the enzymes that break down cartilage. It plays a role in the production of new cartilage.

Benefits of Glucosamine and Chondroitin

✦ Provide relief from symptoms

✦ Reduce pain and tenderness

✦ Reduce swelling

✦ Stimulate the production of cartilage

✦ Improve mobility

As with any other-the-counter products, please check with your doctor before taking any supplements.

Acupuncture. Some people have found pain relief using acupuncture (the use of fine needles inserted at specific points on the skin). Preliminary research shows that acupuncture may be a useful component in an osteoarthritis treatment plan for some patients.

Folk remedies. Some patients seek alternative therapies for their pain and disability. Some of these alternative therapies have included wearing copper bracelets, drinking herbal teas, and taking mud baths. While these practices are not harmful, some can be expensive. They also cause delays in seeking medical treatment. To date, no scientific research shows these approaches to be helpful in treating osteoarthritis.

Nutritional supplements. Nutrients such as glucosamine and chondroitin sulfate have been reported to improve the symptoms of people with osteoarthritis, as have certain vitamins.

Keep a "Good-Health Attitude"

People with osteoarthritis can enjoy good health despite having the disease. How? By learning self-care skills and developing a "good-health attitude."

Self-care is central to successfully managing the pain and disability of osteoarthritis. People have a much better chance of having a rewarding lifestyle when they educate themselves about the disease and take part in their own care. Working actively with a team of health care providers enables people with the disease to minimize pain, share in decision-making about treatment, and feel a sense of control over their lives. Research shows that people with osteoarthritis who take part in their own care report less pain and make fewer doctor visits. They also enjoy a better quality of life.

Self-help and education programs: Three kinds of programs help people learn about osteoarthritis, learn self-care, and improve their good-health attitude. These programs include

- Patient education programs
- Arthritis self-management programs
- Arthritis support groups.

These programs teach people about osteoarthritis, its treatments, exercise and relaxation, patient and health care provider communication, and problem-solving. Research has shown that these programs have clear and long-lasting benefits.

Exercise: Regular physical activity plays a key role in self-care and wellness. You'll read more about this in Part II.

Attitude: Good health also requires a positive attitude. People must decide to make the most of things when faced with the challenges of osteoarthritis. This attitude—a good-health mindset—doesn't just happen. It takes work, every day. And with the right attitude, you will achieve it.

Current Research

The leading role in osteoarthritis research is played by the National Institute of Arthritis and Musculoskeletal and Skin Diseases (NIAMS), within the National Institutes of Health (NIH). The NIAMS funds many researchers across the United States to study osteoarthritis. It has established a Specialized Center of Research devoted to osteoarthritis. Also, many researchers study arthritis at NIAMS Multipurpose Arthritis and Musculoskeletal Diseases Centers and Multidisciplinary Clinical Research Centers. These centers conduct basic, laboratory, and clinical research aimed at understanding the causes, treatment options, and prevention of arthritis and musculoskeletal diseases. Center researchers also study epidemiology, health services, and professional, patient, and public education. The NIAMS also supports multidisciplinary clinical research centers that expand clinical studies for diseases like osteoarthritis.

For years, scientists thought that osteoarthritis was simply a disease of "wear and tear" that occurred in joints as people got older. In the last decade, however, research has shown that there is more to the disorder than aging alone. The production, maintenance, and breakdown of cartilage, as well as bone changes in osteoarthritis, are now seen as a series or cascade of events. Many researchers are trying to discover where in that cascade of events things go wrong. By understanding what goes wrong, they hope to find new ways to prevent or treat osteoarthritis. Some key areas of research are described below.

Self-Management Programs Help

People with osteoarthritis find that self-management programs help them

+ Understand the disease

+ Reduce pain while remaining active

+ Cope physically, emotionally, and mentally

+ Have greater control over the disease

+ Build confidence in their ability to live an active, independent life.

Enjoy a "Good-Health Attitude"

✦ Focus on your abilities instead of disabilities.

✦ Focus on your strengths instead of weaknesses.

✦ Break down activities into small tasks that you can manage.

✦ Incorporate fitness and nutrition into daily routines.

✦ Develop methods to minimize and manage stress.

✦ Balance rest with activity.

✦ Develop a support system of family, friends, and health professionals.

Animal models. Animals help researchers understand how diseases work and why they occur. Animal models help researchers learn many things about osteoarthritis, such as what happens to cartilage, how treatment strategies might work, and what might prevent the disease. Animal models also help scientists study osteoarthritis in very early stages before it causes detectable joint damage.

Some scientists want to find ways to detect osteoarthritis at earlier stages so that they can treat it earlier. They seek specific abnormalities in the blood, joint fluid, or urine of people with the disease. Other scientists use new technologies to analyze the differences between the cartilage from different joints. For example, many people have osteoarthritis in the knees or hips, but few have it in the ankles. Can ankle cartilage be different? Does it age differently? Answering these questions will help us understand the disease better.

Genetics studies. Researchers suspect that inheritance plays a role in 25 to 30 percent of osteoarthritis cases. Researchers have found that genetics may play a role in approximately 40 to 65 percent of hand and knee osteoarthritis cases. They suspect inheritance might play a role in other types of osteoarthritis, as well. Scientists have identified a mutation (a gene defect) affecting collagen, an important part of cartilage, in patients with an inherited kind of osteoarthritis that starts at an early age. The mutation weakens collagen protein, which may break or tear more easily under stress. Scientists are looking for other gene mutations in osteoarthritis. Recently, researchers found that the daughters of women who have knee osteoarthritis have a significant increase in cartilage breakdown, thus making them more susceptible to disease. In the future, a test to determine who carries the genetic defect (or defects) could help people reduce their risk for osteoarthritis with lifestyle adjustments.

Tissue engineering. This technology involves removing cells from a healthy part of the body and placing them in an area of diseased or damaged tissue in order to improve certain body functions. Currently, it is used to treat small traumatic injuries or defects in cartilage, and, if successful, could eventually help treat osteoarthritis. Researchers at the NIAMS are exploring three types of tissue engineering. The two most common methods being studied today include cartilage cell replacement and stem cell transplantation. The third method is gene therapy.

Cartilage cell replacement. In this procedure, researchers remove cartilage cells from the patient's own joint and then clone or grow new cells using tissue culture and other laboratory techniques. They then inject the newly grown cells into the patient's joint. Patients with cartilage cell replacement have fewer symptoms of osteoarthritis. Actual cartilage repair is limited, however.

Stem cell transplantation. Stem cells are primitive cells that can transform into other kinds of cells, such as muscle or bone cells. They usually are taken from bone marrow. In the future, researchers hope to insert stem cells into cartilage, where the cells will make new cartilage. If successful, this process could be used to repair damaged cartilage and avoid the need for surgical joint replacements with metal or plastics.

Gene therapy. Scientists are working to genetically engineer cells that would inhibit the body chemicals, called enzymes, that may help break down cartilage and cause joint damage. In gene therapy, cells are removed from the body, genetically changed, and then injected back into the affected joint. They live in the joint and protect it from damaging enzymes.

Comprehensive treatment strategies. Effective treatment for osteoarthritis takes more than medicine or surgery. Getting help from a variety of care professionals often can improve patient treatment and self-care. Research shows that adding patient education and social support is a low-cost, effective way to decrease pain and reduce the amount of medicine used.

Exercise plays a key part in comprehensive treatment. Researchers are studying exercise in greater detail and finding out just how to use it in treating or preventing osteoarthritis. For example, several scientists have studied knee osteoarthritis and exercise. Their results included the following:

* Strengthening the thigh muscle (quadriceps) can relieve symptoms of knee osteoarthritis and prevent more damage.

* Walking can result in better functioning, and the more you walk, the farther you will be able to walk.

✦ People with knee osteoarthritis who were active in an exercise program feel less pain. They also function better.

Research has shown that losing extra weight can help people who already have osteoarthritis. Moreover, overweight or obese people who do not have osteoarthritis may reduce their risk of developing the disease by losing weight.

Using NSAIDs. Many people who have osteoarthritis have persistent pain despite taking simple pain relievers such as acetaminophen. Some of these patients take NSAIDs instead. Health care providers are concerned about long-term NSAID use because it can lead to an upset stomach, heartburn, nausea, and more dangerous side effects, such as ulcers.

Scientists are working to design and test new, safer NSAIDs. One example currently available is a class of selective NSAIDs called COX-2 inhibitors. Traditional NSAIDs prevent inflammation by blocking two related enzymes in the body called COX-1 and COX-2. The gastrointestinal side effects associated with traditional NSAIDs seems to be associated mainly with blocking the COX-1 enzyme, which helps protect the stomach lining. The new selective COX-2 inhibitors, however, primarily block the COX-2 enzyme, which helps control inflammation in the body. As a result, COX-2 inhibitors reduce pain and inflammation but are less likely than traditional NSAIDs to cause gastrointestinal ulcers and bleeding. However, research shows that some COX-2 inhibitors may not protect against heart disease as well as traditional NSAIDs, so check with your doctor if you have concerns.

Drugs to prevent joint damage. No treatment actually prevents osteoarthritis or reverses or blocks the disease process once it begins. Present treatments just relieve the symptoms. Researchers are looking for drugs that would prevent, slow down, or reverse joint damage. One experimental antibiotic drug, doxycycline, may stop certain enzymes from damaging cartilage. The drug has shown some promise in clinical studies, but more studies are needed. Researchers also are studying growth factors and other natural chemical messengers. These potential medicines may be able to stimulate cartilage growth or repair.

Acupuncture. During an acupuncture treatment, a licensed acupuncture therapist inserts very fine needles into the skin at various points on the body. Scientists think the needles stimulate the release of natural, pain-relieving chemicals produced by the brain or the nervous system. Researchers are studying acupuncture treatment of patients who have knee osteoarthritis. Early findings suggest that traditional Chinese acupuncture is effective for some patients as an additional therapy for osteoarthritis, reducing pain and improving function.

Nutritional supplements. Nutritional supplements are often reported as helpful in treating osteoarthritis. Such reports should be viewed with caution, however, since very few studies have carefully evaluated the role of nutritional supplements in osteoarthritis.

Glucosamine and chondroitin sulfate. Both of these nutrients are found in small quantities in food and are components of normal cartilage. Scientific studies on these two nutritional supplements have not yet shown that they affect the disease. They may relieve symptoms and reduce joint damage in some patients, however. The National Center for Complementary and Alternative Medicine at the NIH is supporting a clinical trial to test whether glucosamine, chondroitin sulfate, or the two nutrients in combination reduce pain and improve function. Patients using this therapy should do so only under the supervision of their doctor, as part of an overall treatment program with exercise, relaxation, and pain relief.

Vitamins D, C, E, and beta carotene. The progression of osteoarthritis may be slower in people who take higher levels of vitamin D, C, E, or beta carotene. More studies are needed to confirm these reports.

Hyaluronic acid. Injecting this substance into the knee joint provides long-term pain relief for some people with osteoarthritis. Hyaluronic acid is a natural component of cartilage and joint fluid. It lubricates and absorbs shock in the joint. The Food and Drug Administration (FDA) approved this therapy for patients with osteoarthritis of the knee who do not get relief from exercise, physical therapy, or simple analgesics. Researchers are presently studying the benefits of using hyaluronic acid to treat osteoarthritis.

Estrogen. In studies of older women, scientists found a lower risk of osteoarthritis in women who had used oral estrogens for hormone replacement therapy. The researchers suspect having low levels of estrogen could increase the risk of developing osteoarthritis. Additional studies are needed to answer this question.

Hope for the Future

Research is opening up new avenues of treatment for people with osteoarthritis. A balanced, comprehensive approach is still the key to staying active and healthy with the disease. People with osteoarthritis should combine exercise, relaxation education, social support, and medicines in their treatment strategies. Meanwhile, as scientists unravel the complexities of the disease, new treatments and prevention methods should appear. They will improve the quality of life for people with osteoarthritis and their families.

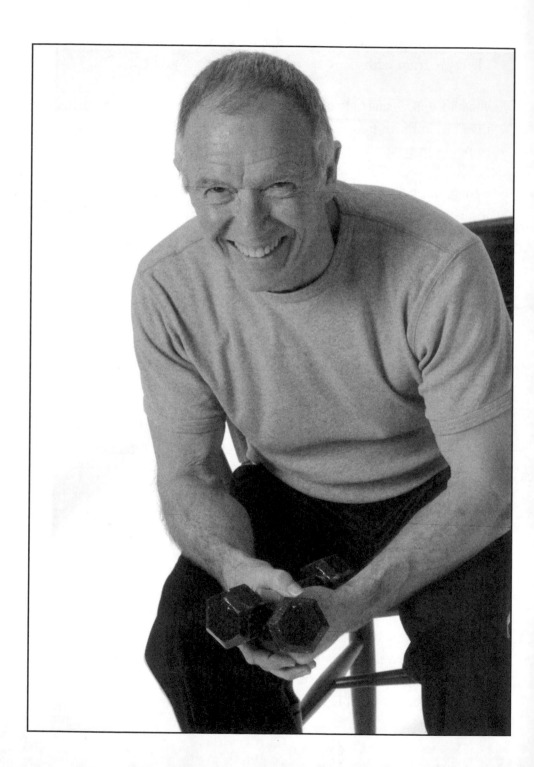

3

Rheumatoid Arthritis

Rheumatoid arthritis is an inflammatory disease that causes pain, swelling, stiffness, and loss of function in the joints. It has several special features that make it different from other kinds of arthritis (see Features of Rheumatoid Arthritis, page 33). For example, rheumatoid arthritis generally occurs in a symmetrical pattern. This means that if one knee or hand is involved, the other one is also. The disease often affects the wrist joints and the finger joints closest to the hand. It can also affect other parts of the body besides the joints (see illustrations below). In addition, people with the disease may have fatigue, occasional fever, and a general sense of not feeling well (malaise).

Another feature of rheumatoid arthritis is that it varies a lot from person to person. For some people, it lasts only a few months or a year or two and goes away without causing any noticeable damage. Other people have mild or moderate disease, with periods of worsening symptoms, called flares, and periods in which they feel

Normal Joint

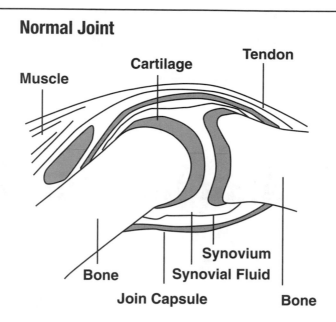

Muscle

Cartilage

Tendon

Bone

Synovium

Synovial Fluid

Join Capsule

Bone

Joint Affected by Rheumatoid Arthritis

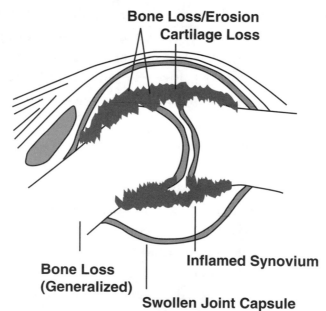

Bone Loss/Erosion

Cartilage Loss

Bone Loss (Generalized)

Inflamed Synovium

Swollen Joint Capsule

Features of Rheumatoid Arthritis

- Tender, warm, swollen joints.

- Symmetrical pattern. For example, if one knee is affected, the other one is also.

- Joint inflammation often affecting the wrist and finger joints closest to the hand; other affected joints can include those of the neck, shoulders, elbows, hips, knees, ankles, and feet.

- Fatigue, occasional fever, a general sense of not feeling well (malaise).

- Pain and stiffness lasting for more than 30 minutes in the morning or after a long rest.

- Symptoms that can last for many years.

- Symptoms in other parts of the body besides the joints.

- Variability of symptoms among people with the disease.

better, called remissions. Still others have severe disease that is active most of the time, lasts for many years, and leads to serious joint damage and disability.

Although rheumatoid arthritis can have serious effects on a person's life and well-being, current treatment strategies—including pain relief and other medications, a balance between rest and exercise, and patient education and support programs—allow most people with the disease to lead active and productive lives. In recent years, research has led to a new understanding of rheumatoid arthritis and has increased the likelihood that, in time, researchers can find ways to greatly reduce the impact of this disease.

How Rheumatoid Arthritis Develops and Progresses

The Joints

A normal joint (the place where two bones meet) is surrounded by a joint capsule that protects and supports it (see illustration on page 32). Cartilage covers and cushions the ends of the two bones. The joint capsule is lined with a type of tissue called synovium, which produces synovial fluid. This clear fluid lubricates and nourishes the cartilage and bones inside the joint capsule.

In rheumatoid arthritis, the immune system, for unknown reasons, attacks a person's own cells inside the joint capsule. White blood cells that are part of the normal immune system travel to the synovium and cause a reaction. This reaction, or inflammation, is called synovitis, and it results in the warmth, redness, swelling, and pain that are typical symptoms of rheumatoid arthritis. During the inflammation process, the cells of the synovium grow and divide abnormally, making the normally thin synovium thick and resulting in a joint that is swollen and puffy to the touch (see illustration).

As rheumatoid arthritis progresses, these abnormal synovial cells begin to invade and destroy the cartilage and bone within the joint. The surrounding muscles, ligaments, and tendons that support and stabilize the joint become weak and unable to work normally. All of these effects lead to the pain and deformities often seen in rheumatoid arthritis. Doctors studying rheumatoid arthritis now believe that damage to bones begins during the first year or two that a person has the disease. This is one reason early diagnosis and treatment are so important in the management of rheumatoid arthritis.

A joint (the place where two bones meet) is surrounded by a capsule that protects and supports it. The joint capsule is lined with a type of tissue called synovium, which produces synovial fluid that lubricates and nourishes joint tissues. In rheumatoid arthritis, the synovium becomes inflamed, causing warmth, redness, swelling, and pain. As the disease progresses, abnormal synovial cells invade and erode, or destroy, cartilage and bone within the joint. Surrounding muscles, ligaments, and tendons become weakened. Rheumatoid arthritis can also cause more generalized bone loss that may lead to osteoporosis (fragile bones that are prone to fracture).

Other Parts of the Body

Some people also experience the effects of rheumatoid arthritis in places other than the joints. About one-quarter develop rheumatoid nodules. These are bumps under the skin that often form close to the joints. Many people with rheumatoid arthritis develop anemia, or a decrease in the normal number of red blood cells. Other effects, which occur less often, include neck pain and dry eyes and mouth. Very rarely, people may have inflammation of the blood vessels, the lining of the lungs, or the sac enclosing the heart.

Occurrence and Impact of Rheumatoid Arthritis

Scientists estimate that about 2.1 million people, or 1 percent of the U.S. adult population, have rheumatoid arthritis. Interestingly, some recent studies have suggested that the overall number of new cases of rheumatoid arthritis may actually be going down. Scientists are now investigating why this may be happening.

Rheumatoid arthritis occurs in all races and ethnic groups. Although the disease often begins in middle age and occurs with increased frequency in older people, children and young adults also develop it. Like some other forms of arthritis, rheumatoid arthritis occurs much more frequently in women than in men. About two to three times as many women as men have the disease.

By all measures, the financial and social impact of all types of arthritis, including rheumatoid arthritis, is substantial, both for the nation and for individuals. From an economic standpoint, the medical and surgical treatment for rheumatoid arthritis and the wages lost because of disability caused by the disease add up to millions of dollars. Daily joint pain is an inevitable consequence of the disease, and most patients also experience some degree of depression, anxiety, and feelings of helplessness. In some cases, rheumatoid arthritis can interfere with a person's ability to carry out normal daily activities, limit job opportunities, or disrupt the joys and responsibilities of family life. However, there are arthritis self-management programs that help people cope with the pain and other effects of the disease and help them lead independent and productive lives. These programs are described later in the section Diagnosing and Treating Rheumatoid Arthritis.

Searching for the Cause of Rheumatoid Arthritis

Rheumatoid arthritis is one of several "autoimmune" diseases ("auto" means self), so-called because a person's immune system attacks his or her own body tissues. Scientists still do not know exactly what causes this to happen, but research over the last few years has begun to unravel the factors involved.

Genetic (inherited) factors. Scientists have found that certain genes that play a role in the immune system are associated with a tendency to develop rheumatoid arthritis. At the same time, some people with rheumatoid arthritis do not have these particular genes, and other people have these genes but never develop the disease. This suggests that a person's genetic makeup is an important part of the story but not the whole answer. It is clear, however, that more than one gene is involved in determining whether a person develops rheumatoid arthritis and, if so, how severe the disease will become.

Environmental factors. Many scientists think that something must occur to trigger the disease process in people whose genetic make-up makes them susceptible to rheumatoid arthritis. An infectious agent such as a virus or bacterium appears likely, but the exact agent is not yet known. Note, however, that rheumatoid arthritis is not contagious: A person cannot "catch" it from someone else.

Other factors. Some scientists also think that a variety of hormonal factors may be involved. These hormones, or possibly deficiencies or changes in certain hormones, may promote the development of rheumatoid arthritis in a genetically susceptible person who has been exposed to a triggering agent from the environment.

Even though all the answers aren't known, one thing is certain: Rheumatoid arthritis develops as a result of an interaction of many factors. Much research is going on now to understand these factors and how they work together.

Diagnosing and Treating Rheumatoid Arthritis

Diagnosing and treating rheumatoid arthritis is a team effort between the patient and several types of health care professionals. A person can go to his or her family doctor or internist or to a rheumatologist. A rheumatologist is a doctor who specializes in arthritis and other diseases of the joints, bones, and muscles. As treatment progresses, other professionals often help. These may include nurses, physical or occupational therapists, orthopedic surgeons, psychologists, and social workers.

Studies have shown that people who are well informed and participate actively in their own care experience less pain and make fewer visits to the doctor than do other people with rheumatoid arthritis.

Patient education and arthritis self-management programs, as well as support groups, help people to become better informed and to participate in their own care. An example of a self-management program is the arthritis self-help course offered by the Arthritis Foundation and developed at one of the NIAMS-supported Multipurpose Arthritis and Musculoskeletal Diseases Centers. Self-management programs teach about rheumatoid arthritis and its treatments, exercise and relaxation approaches, patient/health care provider communication, and problem solving. Research on these programs has shown that they have the following clear and long-lasting benefits:

+ They help people understand the disease.

+ They help people reduce their pain while remaining active.

+ They help people cope physically, emotionally, and mentally.

+ They help people feel greater control over their disease and help build a sense of confidence in the ability to function and lead a full, active, and independent life.

Diagnosis

Early diagnosis of rheumatoid arthritis is important. People who have early stage RA and receive aggressive care have better outcomes, improvement in the arthritis and physical function and less joint damage. But rheumatoid arthritis can be difficult to diagnose in its early stages for several reasons. First, there is no single test for the disease. In addition, symptoms differ from person to person. Also, symptoms can be similar to those of other types of arthritis and joint conditions, and it may take time for other conditions to be ruled out.

Finally, the full range of symptoms develops over time; only a few may be present in the early stages. As a result, doctors use a variety of tools to diagnose the disease and to rule out other conditions.

Medical history. This is the patient's description of symptoms and when and how they began. Good communication between patient and doctor is especially important here. For example, the patient's description of pain, stiffness, and joint function and how these change over time is critical to the doctor's initial assessment of the disease and his or her assessment of how the disease changes.

Physical examination. This includes the doctor's examination of the joints, skin, reflexes, and muscle strength.

Laboratory tests. One common test is for rheumatoid factor, an antibody that is eventually present in the blood of most rheumatoid arthritis patients. (An antibody is a special protein made by the immune system that normally helps fight foreign substances in the body.) Not all people with rheumatoid arthritis test positive for rheumatoid factor, however, especially early in the disease. And, some others who do test positive never develop the disease. Other common tests include one that indicates the presence of inflammation in the body (the erythrocyte sedimentation rate), a white blood cell count, and a blood test for anemia.

X rays. X rays are used to determine the degree of joint destruction. They are not useful in the early stages of rheumatoid arthritis before bone damage is evident, but they can be used later to monitor the progression of the disease.

Treatment

Doctors use a variety of approaches to treat rheumatoid arthritis. These are used in different combinations and at different times during the course of the disease and are chosen according to the patient's individual situation. No matter what treatment the doctor and patient choose, however, the goals are the same: relieve pain, reduce inflammation, slow down or stop joint damage, and improve the person's sense of well-being and ability to function.

Treatment is another key area for communication between patient and doctor. Talking to the doctor can help ensure that exercise and pain management programs are provided as needed and that drugs are prescribed appropriately. Talking can also help in making decisions about surgery.

Lifestyle

This approach includes several activities that help improve a person's ability to function independently and maintain a positive outlook.

Rest and exercise. Both rest and exercise help in important ways. People with rheumatoid arthritis need a good balance between the two, with more rest when the disease is active and more exercise when it is not. Rest helps to reduce active joint inflammation and pain and to fight fatigue. The length of time needed for rest will vary from person to person, but in general, shorter rest breaks every now and then are more helpful than long times spent in bed.

Exercise, is important for maintaining healthy and strong muscles, preserving joint mobility, and maintaining flexibility. Exercise can also help people sleep well, reduce pain, maintain a positive attitude, and lose weight. Exercise programs should be planned and carried out to take into account the person's physical abilities, limitations, and changing needs.

Goals of Treatment

+ Relieve pain
+ Reduce inflammation
+ Slow down or stop joint damage
+ Improve a person's sense of well-being and ability to function

Current Treatment Approaches

+ Lifestyle
+ Medications
+ Surgery
+ Routine monitoring and ongoing care

Care of joints. Some people find that using a splint for a short time around a painful joint reduces pain and swelling by supporting the joint and letting it rest. Splints are used mostly on wrists and hands, but also on ankles and feet. A doctor or a physical or occupational therapist can help a patient get a splint and ensure that it fits properly. Other ways to reduce stress on joints include self-help devices (for example, zipper pullers, long-handled shoe horns); devices to help with getting on and off chairs, toilet seats, and beds; and changes in the ways that a person carries out daily activities.

Stress reduction. People with rheumatoid arthritis face emotional challenges as well as physical ones. The emotions they feel because of the disease—fear, anger, frustration—combined with any pain and physical limitations can increase their stress level. Although there is no evidence that stress plays a role in causing rheumatoid arthritis, it can make living with the disease difficult at times. Stress may also affect the amount of pain a person feels. There are a number of successful techniques for coping with stress. Regular rest periods can help, as can relaxation, distraction, or visualization exercises. Exercise programs, participation in support groups, and good communication with the health care team are other ways to reduce stress.

Healthful diet. With the exception of several specific types of oils, there is no scientific evidence that any specific food or nutrient helps or harms most people with rheumatoid arthritis. However, an overall nutritious diet with enough—but not an excess of—calories, protein, and calcium is important. Some people may need to be careful about drinking alcoholic beverages because of the medications they take for rheumatoid arthritis. Those taking methotrexate may need to avoid alcohol altogether. Patients should ask their doctors for guidance on this issue.

Climate. Some people notice that their arthritis gets worse when there is a sudden change in the weather. However, there is no evidence that a specific climate can prevent or reduce the effects of rheumatoid arthritis. Moving to a new place with a different climate usually does not make a long-term difference in a person's rheumatoid arthritis.

Medications

Most people who have rheumatoid arthritis take medications. Some medications are used only for pain relief; others are used to reduce inflammation. Still others—often called disease-modifying antirheumatic drugs, or DMARDs—are used to try to slow the course of the disease. The person's general condition, the current and predicted severity of the illness, the length of time he or she will take the drug, and the drug's effectiveness and potential side effects are important considerations in prescribing drugs for rheumatoid arthritis. The table on pages 44 and 45 about "Medications Commonly Used To Treat Rheumatoid Arthritis" shows currently used rheumatoid arthritis medications, along with their effects, side effects, and monitoring requirements.

Traditionally, rheumatoid arthritis therapy has involved an approach in which doctors prescribed aspirin or similar drugs, rest, and physical therapy first, and prescribed more powerful drugs later only if the disease became much worse. Recently, many doctors have changed their approach, especially for patients with severe, rapidly progressing rheumatoid arthritis. This change is based on the belief that early treatment with more powerful drugs, and the use of drug combinations in place of single drugs, may be more effective ways to halt the progression of the disease and reduce or prevent joint damage.

Surgery

Several types of surgery are available to patients with severe joint damage. The primary purpose of these procedures is to reduce pain, improve the affected joint's function, and improve the patient's ability to perform daily activities. Surgery is not for everyone, however, and the decision should be made only after careful consideration by patient and doctor. Together they should discuss the patient's overall health, the condition of the joint or tendon that will be operated on, and the reason for and the risks and benefits of, the surgical procedure. Cost may be another factor. Commonly performed surgical procedures include joint replacement, tendon reconstruction, and synovectomy.

Joint replacement. This is the most frequently performed surgery for rheumatoid arthritis, and it is done primarily to relieve pain and improve or preserve joint function. Artificial joints are not always

Medications Commonly Used to Treat Rheumatoid Arthritis

Aspirin and other non-steroidal anti-inflammatory drugs (NSAIDs)

- Used to reduce pain, swelling, and inflammation, allowing patients to move more easily and carry out normal activities.
- Generally part of early and continuing therapy.

Drug Name	Manufacturer	Generic Name
Actron	Bayer	ketoprofen
Advil	Wyeth	ibuprofen
Aleve	Bayer	naproxen
Buffered Aspirin	Various	buffered aspirin
Celebrex	Pfizer	celecoxib
Motrin IB	McNeil Consumer	ibuprofen
Naprosyn	Roche Laboratories	naproxen
Nuprin	Bristol-Myers Squibb	ibuprofen
Orudis	Wyeth	ketoprofen
Plain Aspirin	Various	aspirin
Vioxx	Merck	rofecoxib

Disease-modifying antirheumatic drugs (DMARDs)—also called slow-acting antirheumatic drugs (SAARDs) or second-line drugs.

- Used to alter the course of the disease and prevent joint and cartilage destruction.
- May produce significant improvement for many patients.
- Exactly how they work still unknown.
- Generally take a few weeks or months to have an effect.
- Patients may use several over the course of the disease.

Drug Name	Manufacturer	Generic Name
Azulfidine	Pharmacia and Upjohn	sulfasalazine
Cuprimine	Merck	penicillamine
Plaquenil	Sanofi-Synthelabo	hydroxychloroquine sulfate
Ridaura	Prometheus Laboratories	auranofin

Immunosuppresants (also considered DMARDs)

- Used to restrain the overly active immune system, which is key to the disease process.
- Same concerns as with other DMARDs: potential toxicity and diminishing effectiveness over time.

Drug Name	Manufacturer	Generic Name
Arava	Aventis	leflunomide
Azasan	AAI Pharma	azathioprine
Neoral	Novartis	cyclosporine
Rheumatrex	Stada	methotrexate sodium
Sandimmune	Novartis	cyclosporine

Corticosteroids (also known as glucocorticoids)

- Used for their anti-inflammatory and immunosuppressive effects.
- Given either in pill form or an injection into a joint.
- Dramatic improvements in a very short time.
- Potential for serious side effects, especially at high doses.
- Often used early while waiting for DMARDs to work.
- Also used for severe flares and when the disease does not respond to NSAIDs and DMARDs.

Drug Name	Manufacturer	Generic Name
Deltasone	Pharmacia and Upjohn	prednisone
Medrol	Pharmacia and Upjohn	methylprednisolone

Biologic Response Modifiers

- Effective in patients with mild to moderate rheumatoid arthritis who have failed other drug therapies and, in addition, in patients with juvenile rheumatoid arthritis. Give as a twice-a-week injection into the skin.

Drug Name	Manufacturer	Generic Name
Enbrel	Amgen	etanercept

permanent and may eventually have to be replaced. This may be an issue for younger people.

Tendon reconstruction. Rheumatoid arthritis can damage and even rupture tendons, the tissues that attach muscle to bone. This surgery, which is used most frequently on the hands, reconstructs the damaged tendon by attaching an intact tendon to it. This procedure can help to restore hand function, especially if the tendon is completely ruptured.

Synovectomy. In this surgery, the doctor actually removes the inflamed synovial tissue. Synovectomy by itself is seldom performed now because not all of the tissue can be removed, and it eventually grows back. Synovectomy is done as part of reconstructive surgery, especially tendon reconstruction.

Routine Monitoring and Ongoing Care

Regular medical care is important to monitor the course of the disease, determine the effectiveness and any negative effects of medications, and change therapies as needed. Monitoring typically includes regular visits to the doctor. It may also include blood, urine, and other laboratory tests and X rays.

Osteoporosis prevention is one issue that patients may want to discuss with their doctors as part of their long-term, ongoing care. Osteoporosis is a condition in which bones lose calcium and become weakened and fragile. Many older women are at increased risk for osteoporosis, and their rheumatoid arthritis increases the risk further, particularly if they are taking corticosteroids such as prednisone. These patients may want to discuss with their doctors the potential benefits of calcium and vitamin D supplements, hormone replacement therapy, or other treatments for osteoporosis.

Alternative and Complementary Therapies

Special diets, vitamin supplements, and other alternative approaches have been suggested for the treatment of rheumatoid arthritis. Although many of these approaches may not be harmful in and of themselves, controlled scientific studies either have not been conducted or have found no definite benefit to these therapies. Some alternative or complementary approaches may help the patient cope or reduce some of the stress associated with living with a chronic illness. As with any therapy, patients should discuss the benefits and drawbacks with their doctors before beginning an alternative or new type of therapy. If the doctor feels the approach has value and will not be harmful, it can be incorporated into a patient's treatment plan. However, it is important not to neglect regular health care. The Arthritis Foundation publishes material on alternative therapies as well as established therapies, and patients may want to contact this organization for information.

Current Research

Over the last several decades, research has greatly increased our understanding of immunology, genetics, and cellular and molecular biology. This foundation in basic science is now showing results in several areas important to rheumatoid arthritis. Scientists are thinking about rheumatoid arthritis in exciting ways that were not possible even 10 years ago.

The National Institutes of Health funds a wide variety of medical research at its headquarters in Bethesda, Maryland, and at universities and medical centers across the United States. One of the NIH institutes, the National Institute of Arthritis and Musculoskeletal and Skin Diseases, is a major supporter of research and research training in rheumatoid arthritis through grants to individual scientists, specialized centers of research, and multipurpose arthritis and musculoskeletal diseases centers.

Following are examples of current research directions in rheumatoid arthritis supported by the Federal Government through the NIAMS and other parts of the NIH.

Scientists are looking at basic abnormalities in the immune systems of people with rheumatoid arthritis and in some animal models of the disease to understand why and how the disease develops. Findings from these studies may lead to precise, targeted therapies that could stop the inflammatory process in its earliest stages. They may even lead to a vaccine that could prevent rheumatoid arthritis.

Researchers are studying genetic factors that predispose some people to developing rheumatoid arthritis, as well as factors connected with disease severity. Findings from these studies should increase our understanding of the disease and will help develop new therapies as well as guide treatment decisions. In a major effort aimed at identifying genes involved in rheumatoid arthritis, the NIH and the Arthritis Foundation have joined together to support the North American Rheumatoid Arthritis Consortium. This group of 12 research centers around the United States is collecting medical information and genetic material from 1,000 families in which two or more siblings have rheumatoid arthritis. It will serve as a national resource for genetic studies of this disease.

Scientists are also gaining insights into the genetic basis of rheumatoid arthritis by studying rats with autoimmune inflammatory arthritis that resembles human disease. NIAMS researchers have identified several genetic regions that affect arthritis susceptibility and severity in these animal models of the disease, and found some striking similarities between rats and humans. Identifying disease genes in rats should provide important new information that may yield clues to the causes of rheumatoid arthritis in humans.

Scientists are studying the complex relationships among the hormonal, nervous, and immune systems in rheumatoid arthritis. For example, they are exploring whether and how the normal changes in the levels of steroid hormones (such as estrogen and testosterone) during a person's lifetime may be related to the development, improvement, or flares of the disease. Scientists are also looking at how these systems interact with environmental and genetic factors. Results from these studies may suggest new treatment strategies.

Researchers are exploring why so many more women than men develop rheumatoid arthritis. In hopes of finding clues, they are studying female and male hormones and other elements that differ between women and men, such as possible differences in their immune responses.

To find clues to new treatments, researchers are examining why rheumatoid arthritis often improves during pregnancy. Results of one study suggest that the explanation may be related to differences in certain special proteins between a mother and her unborn child. These proteins help the immune system distinguish between the body's own cells and foreign cells. Such differences, the scientists speculate, may change the activity of the mother's immune system during pregnancy.

A growing body of evidence indicates that infectious agents, such as viruses and bacteria, may trigger rheumatoid arthritis in people who have an inherited predisposition to the disease. Investigators are trying to discover which infectious agents may be responsible. More broadly, they are also working to understand the basic mechanisms by which these agents might trigger the development of rheumatoid arthritis. Identifying the agents and understanding how they work could lead to new therapies.

Scientists are searching for new drugs or combinations of drugs that can reduce inflammation, can slow or stop the progression of rheumatoid arthritis, and also have few side effects. Studies in humans have shown that a number of compounds have such potential. For example, some studies are breaking new ground in the area of "biopharmaceuticals," or "biologics." These new drugs are based on compounds occurring naturally in the body, and are designed to target specific aspects of the inflammatory process.

Investigators have also shown that treatment of rheumatoid arthritis with minocycline, a drug in the tetracycline family, has a modest benefit. The effects of a related tetracycline called doxycycline are under investigation. Other studies have shown that the omega-3 fatty acids in certain fish or plant seed oils also may reduce rheumatoid arthritis inflammation. However, many people are not able to tolerate the large amounts of oil necessary for any benefit.

Investigators are examining many issues related to quality of life for rheumatoid arthritis patients and quality, cost, and effectiveness of health care services for these patients. Scientists have found that even a small improvement in a patient's sense of physical and mental well-being can have an impact on his or her quality of life and use of health care services. Results from studies like these will help health care providers design integrated treatment strategies that cover all of a patient's needs—emotional as well as physical.

Results of Recent Studies

Patients with early stage rheumatoid arthritis (RA) showed significantly greater improvement when treated with doxycycline plus methotrexate.

*   Positive results were seen in patients with severe RA who were treated with alefacept plus methotrexate. Alefacept is a biologic drug that selectively depletes memory-effector T cells. T cells are involved in cellular immune responses.

*   A new blood test can identify people at very high risk for RA. Early detection and treatment can prevent a chronic, disabling disease.

*   Interleukin-1, used to manage RA, may also be safe and effective in managing osteoarthritis.

From "Clinical Update in Musculoskeletal Medicine. RA and Related Rheumatoid Conditions: The Latest Advances." *The Journal of Musculoskeletal Medicine.* December 2003.

Hope for the Future

Scientists are making rapid progress in understanding the complexities of rheumatoid arthritis—how and why it develops, why some people get it and others do not, why some people get it more severely than others. Results from research are having an impact today, enabling people with rheumatoid arthritis to remain active in life, family, and work far longer than was possible 20 years ago. There is also hope for tomorrow, as researchers continue to explore ways of stopping the disease process early, before it becomes destructive, or even preventing rheumatoid arthritis altogether.

4

Fibromyalgia

Fibromyalgia is a chronic disorder characterized by widespread musculoskeletal pain, fatigue, and multiple tender points. "Tender points" refers to tenderness that occurs in precise, localized areas, particularly in the neck, spine, shoulders, and hips. People with this syndrome may also experience sleep disturbances, morning stiffness, irritable bowel syndrome, anxiety, and other symptoms.

How Many People Have Fibromyalgia?

According to the American College of Rheumatology, fibromyalgia affects 3 to 6 million Americans. It primarily occurs in women of child-bearing age, but children, the elderly, and men can also be affected.

What Causes Fibromyalgia?

Although the cause of fibromyalgia is unknown, researchers have several theories about causes or triggers of the disorder. Some scientists believe that the syndrome may be caused by an injury or trauma. This injury may affect the central nervous system. Fibromyalgia may be associated with changes in muscle metabolism, such as decreased blood flow, causing fatigue and decreased strength. Others believe the syndrome may be triggered by an infectious agent such as a virus in susceptible people, but no such agent has been identified.

How Is Fibromyalgia Diagnosed?

Fibromyalgia is difficult to diagnose because many of the symptoms mimic those of other disorders. The physician reviews the patient's medical history and makes a diagnosis of fibromyalgia based on a history of chronic widespread pain that persists for more than 3 months. The American College of Rheumatology (ACR) has developed criteria for fibromyalgia that physicians can use in diagnosing the disorder. According to ACR criteria, a person is considered to have fibromyalgia if he or she has widespread pain in combination with tenderness in at least 11 of 18 specific tender point sites.

How Is Fibromyalgia Treated?

Treatment of fibromyalgia requires a comprehensive approach. The physician, physical therapist, and patient may all play an active role in the management of fibromyalgia. Studies have shown that aerobic exercise, such as swimming and walking, improves muscle fitness and reduces muscle pain and tenderness. Heat and massage may also give short-term relief. Antidepressant medications may help elevate mood, improve quality of sleep, and relax muscles. Patients with fibromyalgia may benefit from a combination of exercise, medication, physical therapy, and relaxation.

What Research Is Being Conducted on Fibromyalgia?

The National Institute of Arthritis and Musculoskeletal and Skin Diseases (NIAMS) is sponsoring research that will increase understanding of the specific abnormalities that cause and accompany fibromyalgia with the hope of developing better ways to diagnose, treat, and prevent this disorder.

Recent NIAMS studies show that abnormally low levels of the hormone cortisol may be associated with fibromyalgia. At Brigham and Women's Hospital in Boston, Massachusetts, and at the University of Michigan Medical Center in Ann Arbor, researchers are studying regulation of the function of the adrenal gland (which makes cortisol) in fibromyalgia. People whose bodies make inadequate amounts of cortisol experience many of the same symptoms as people with fibromyalgia. It is hoped that these studies will increase understanding about fibromyalgia and may suggest new ways to treat the disorder.

NIAMS research studies are looking at different aspects of the disorder. At the University of Alabama in Birmingham, researchers are concentrating on how specific brain structures are involved in the painful symptoms of fibromyalgia. At George Washington University in Washington, DC, scientists are investigating the causes of a post-Lyme disease syndrome as a model for fibromyalgia. Some patients develop a fibromyalgia-like condition following Lyme disease, an infectious disorder associated with arthritis and other symptoms.

NIAMS-supported research on fibromyalgia also includes several projects at the Institute's Multipurpose Arthritis and Musculoskeletal Diseases Centers. Researchers at these centers are studying individuals who do not seek medical care, but who meet the criteria for fibromyalgia. (Potential subjects are located through advertisements in local newspapers asking for volunteers with widespread pain or aching.) Other studies at the Centers are attempting to uncover better ways to manage the pain associated with the disorder through behavioral interventions such as relaxation training.

In March 1998, NIAMS and several other NIH institutes and offices issued a Request for Proposals to promote research studies of fibromyalgia. As a result of this request, NIAMS and its partners recently funded 15 new fibromyalgia projects totaling more than $3.6 million.

The NIAMS supports and encourages outstanding basic and clinical research that increases the understanding of fibromyalgia. However, much more research needs to be done before fibromyalgia can be successfully treated or prevented.

The Federal Government, in collaboration with researchers, physicians, and private voluntary health organizations, is committed to research efforts that are directed at significantly improving the health of all Americans afflicted with fibromyalgia.

Surgical Treatments: When is Surgery Necessary?

If the pain of arthritis is persistent, and unresponsive to conservative treatment for pain and/or there is advanced erosion of the joints and severe loss of function, surgery may be indicated. Some of the surgical procedures for degenerative arthritis are as follows:

Arthroscopic debridement is a surgical procedure in which a smooth joint surface is created by shaving down the rough edges of the cartilage. The remaining debris is then flushed out of the joint space with saline. The incision is very small. A thin, wand-like lens, attached to a camera, is inserted through the incision. The surgeon is able to "see" the joint by looking on a monitor.

The advantages of arthroscopic, as opposed to an open procedure are: less recovery time, smaller incision, less risk for infection, less post operative pain, reduced complications and a reduced hospital stay.

Arthroplasty, or joint replacement with an artificial joint, is performed to restore motion to the joint and function to the muscles and ligaments. It is indicated when more conservative treatments have failed. Sometimes the entire or only a part of the joint is replaced. Although joint replacement surgery as become refined over the years, and enjoys a high rate of success it is not without complications. Some potential complications are: infection, pulmonary emboli (blood clot), and loosening of the implant. Antibiotics are usually given before surgery to minimize the risk of infection. If you have joint replacement surgery you will be referred to physical therapy. It is important to attend the sessions. There will be certain positions that you should avoid. In the case of hip replacement surgery, you should not flex the hip beyond 90 degrees. In other words, don't bring the knee higher than the operative hip. You should turn the replacement hip/leg inward (pigeon toe) and avoid crossing the operative leg over the opposite leg. These positions and exercises for the hip are outlined in the exercise section of this book.

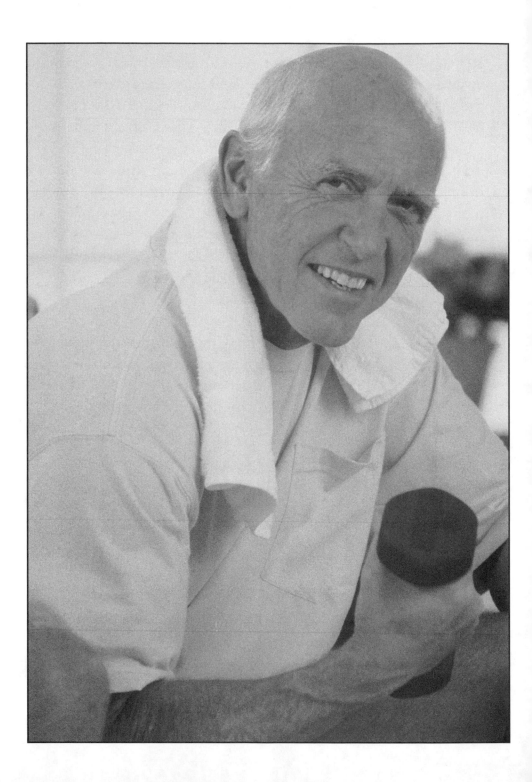

Part II: The Exercises for Arthritis

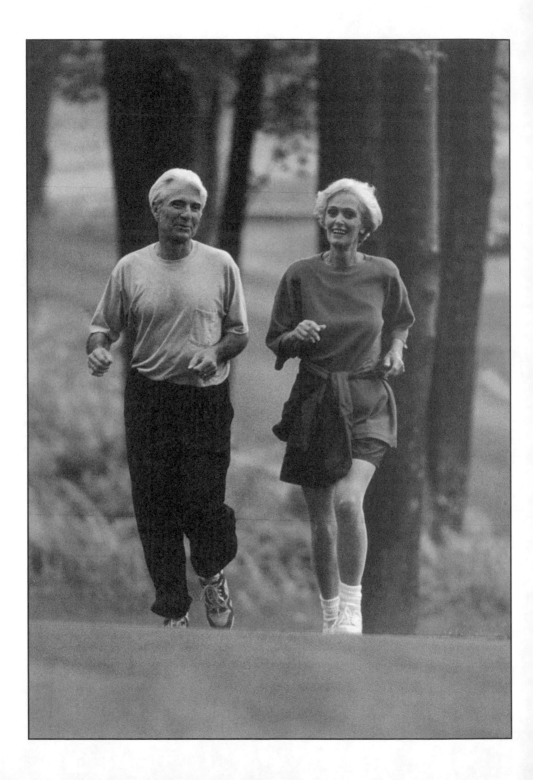

5

Learning to Breathe

Do you ever think about breathing? Probably not. Breathing is automatic; we don't give it much thought. However, many people, especially if they are in pain, tend to take shallow breaths. In other words they breathe from the upper chest. This is a very ineffective way to breathe since the lungs can't fully inflate and take in life-sustaining oxygen. Proper breathing becomes even more critical when you are exercising because your oxygen requirement increases. You need to use your breathing muscles: the diaphragm, stomach and intercostals muscles. The diaphragm performs most of the work in getting air in and out of your lungs. It is below your lungs and separates your chest cavity from your abdomen. It lowers as you inhale and rises as you exhale. The intercostals muscles are located around your rib cage and help the rib cage to expand and contract.

You can strengthen your breathing muscles by practicing diaphragmatic and pursed-lip breathing. You may want to include these breathing exercises in your daily routine of exercises. By learning proper breathing techniques and performing other exercises to make your body strong, you will breathe more efficiently and feel better.

Basic Breathing Exercises

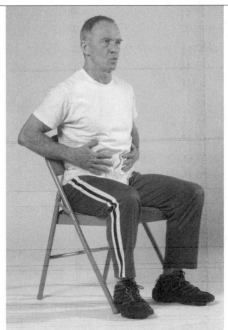

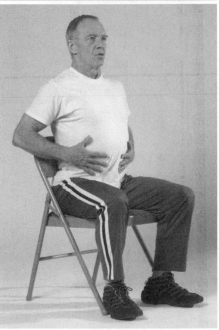

Seated Diaphragmatic Breathing

1. Sit comfortably in a chair with your back straight and supported. Sit upright and with good posture. Align your shoulders over your hips and lift your rib cage away from your hips.

2. Place one hand on your chest to feel the movement of your rib cage.

3. Place the other hand on your upper stomach area to feel the movement of your diaphragm.

4. Pull your stomach muscles in as you exhale slowly through pursed lips (pretend you're blowing out your birthday candles).

5. Inhale through your nose, feeling your stomach muscles relax.

6. Perform 3 to 4 breaths, take a break, and then repeat.

Basic Breathing Exercises

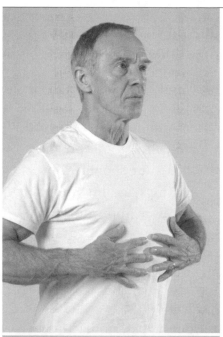

Standing Rib Cage Breathing

1 Stand tall with good posture.

2 Place your hands over your lower ribs.

3 Inhale slowly through your nose, feeling your ribs expand.

4 Feel your lower ribs move down as you exhale through pursed lips.

5 Perform 3 to 4 breaths, take a break and then repeat.

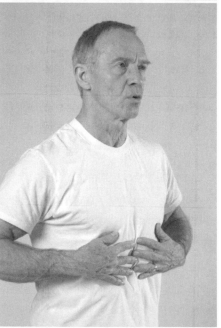

Practice both exercises 2 to 3 times per day. After a while, it will become your normal way of breathing. Whenever you exercise use this breathing technique. Exhale as you do the work part of the exercise and inhale during the preparation phase of the exercise. A bonus is that it will also strengthen your abdominal muscles.

Basic Breathing Exercises

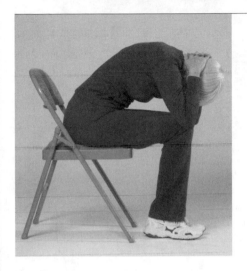

Breathing & Abdominal Strengthening Exercise

This exercise strengthens your abdominal and breathing muscles. Rest between each exercise and lower only to a point that feels comfortable for you.

1. Sit up tall with your back straight against the back of the chair.

2. Place your hands behind your head with your elbows pointed out to the side. Inhale slowly through your nose.

3. As you breathe out slowly through pursed lips, bend slowly bringing your chest toward your thighs. Bring your elbows in toward your face.

4. Inhale as you slowly return to the starting sitting position. Repeat 5 to 7 times.

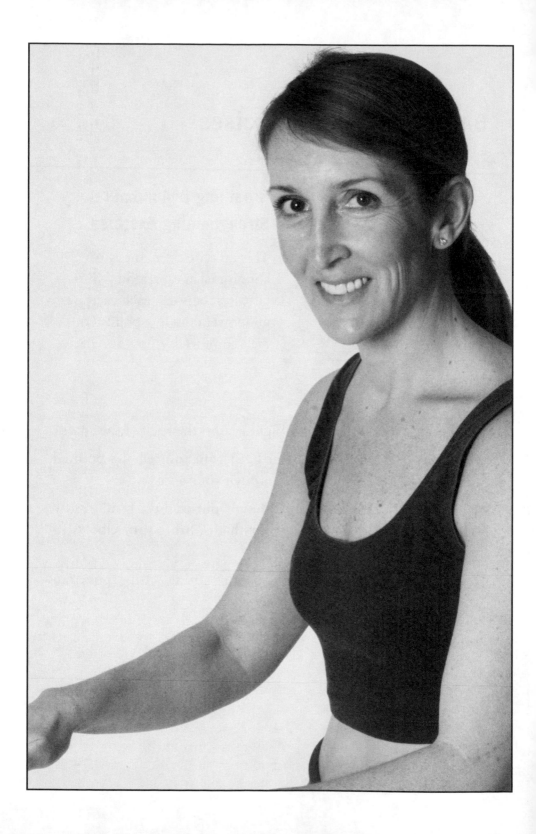

6

Starting an Exercise Program

The hardest part of exercising is getting started. Once you've made the commitment to exercise, make room in your schedule to allow it to happen. Don't get distracted by other chores that need to get done. Focus on your scheduled exercise time and do it! You will feel much better and more energized when you're finished.

Posture and Alignment

It is important to maintain proper posture and body alignment before initiating movement and throughout exercise. When you're not feeling well or are in pain, you might tend to hunch your shoulders and hold your body in a guarded, tense position. Muscle tension can contribute to your discomfort; keeping your body in correct alignment can actually reduce pain. Stand tall, but keep your posture relaxed. Imagine a rod passing from the top of your head through your spine. Hold in your chin and keep your shoulders back, down, and relaxed. Lift and open your chest to allow better expansion of the lungs and improve breathing and oxygenation of the tissues. Pull your abdominal muscles in and tilt your pelvis so the tailbone points downward toward the floor. Avoid arching your back since this places stress on the vertebrae and discs of your spine. Keep your knees soft and slightly bent—don't lock them. Position your feet slightly apart to provide balance and stability.

Warming Up

The benefits of warming up before you work out can't be overemphasized. The warm-up prepares the body for exercise. It provides for a progressive increase in body temperature and circulation, which increases oxygen delivery to the heart. The gradual increase in muscle temperature decreases the risk of injury. The warm-up component of your workout should consist of 5 to 10 minutes of low-intensity activities such as walking, cycling at a slow pace, or light stretching.

About the Exercises

The exercises in this book can be divided into four categories based on their purpose and effects on the body.

+ Range of motion (ROM)

+ Strength training

+ Cardiovascular conditioning

+ Stretching

ROM exercises benefit the joints by encouraging you to move your limbs, head, neck, shoulders, torso, and feet, so the involved joints and surrounding structures can move more freely. The goal is to preserve joint function. Performing ROM exercises upon wakening, even before getting out of bed, will get your blood circulating and ease morning stiffness. I suggest performing ROM exercises on a daily basis. It is a low level exercise that is easily tolerated.

Strength training will improve weight-bearing tolerance and overall function of the muscles and tendons. Isometric exercises are an appropriate mode of strength training as long as the exercises are performed in the pain-free range. Initially, strength exercises can be performed with the weight of the limb moving against gravity. To progressively overload, a necessary ingredient for continuing to develop increasing strength, you can include tubing, exercise bands, or light (1- to 2-pound) ankle or hand weights.

The Arthritis Foundation recommends avoiding strength training during periods of symptom flare-ups and performing fewer rather than more repetitions (the amount of times you perform an exercise).

Pacing Yourself

Exercise is essential for preserving function and strength. Aerobic exercise, such as walking, swimming, and cycling should be comfortably paced. You should exercise at a low to moderate speed.

Use light hand weights or exercise bands to improve strength. Range of motion exercises as outlined in this book will help maintain good joint function. A good rule of thumb is to reduce intensity of the exercise or the amount of time you exercise if you're feeling tired or achy.

Perform 3 to 5 repetitions of an exercise with a rest period between each exercise. It is important to include strength exercises for the gluteus maximus and medius (the buttock and hip muscles) because they help control stability to your back and pelvis. Gait and balance are dependent on having a stable pelvis. This book offers several exercises that will target this area.

Cardiovascular conditioning is important for your overall health. Check with your doctor before beginning this type of exercise because she may want to order a stress test. Recumbent bicycles and steppers, cycling, and walking can strengthen the heart, improve endurance and weight-bearing tolerance as long as they are performed in the pain-free range. Water exercises, such as deep water walking, are beneficial and minimize joint loading forces and joint swelling. It is such a soothing form of exercise—you will love it!

Stretching, the lengthening of the muscle, improves flexibility by allowing your joint to move through its full range of motion without being limited by a shortened muscle and tendon. It can also be very relaxing if you breathe deeply and exhale into the stretch. Continue to take deep breaths as you hold the stretch. When you stretch, you may want to play soft music in the background or light an aromatherapy candle to create a soothing, relaxing atmosphere. It's the perfect way to end the day or to nurture yourself when you need it. The Range of Motion exercises in the next chapter include a stretching component.

General Guidelines for Exercise

+ Never force the joint to move beyond a comfortable range of motion. Be patient: Over time, the range of motion will increase.

+ Keep all movements controlled. Ease in and out of all movements slowly. Be gentle and avoid flinging your limbs.

Tai Chi

Tai chi is a Chinese form of exercise, meditation, and self-defense. It incorporates the philosophy of Taoism, which emphasizes living harmoniously with the environment. By adapting to obstacles and problems rather than taking a confrontational approach, you can flow more evenly through life.

The slow fluid movements of tai chi can help relieve the effects of arthritis, promote flexibility, balance and coordination and develop strength. Tai chi, therefore can be included in all four categories of exercise—range of motion, strength training, cardiovascular conditioning and stretching. The mental relaxation that accompanies the movements of tai chi are beneficial if you experience chronic stress or pain.

To find a local tai chi class, check with local gyms, YMCA, or YWCA.

+ Limit the number of repetitions (the number of times you perform an exercise) to what you can comfortably perform without pain. *Do not* cross the pain threshold. Rest the joint if it is inflamed or painful.

+ Aerobic exercises such as walking, cycling and water exercise will increase your heart function, endurance, lean body mass, and overall health. These are excellent choices for people with arthritis.

+ Choose *your* best time of day to exercise. If you tend to be stiff in the morning or too tired at night, try exercising in the late morning or late afternoon.

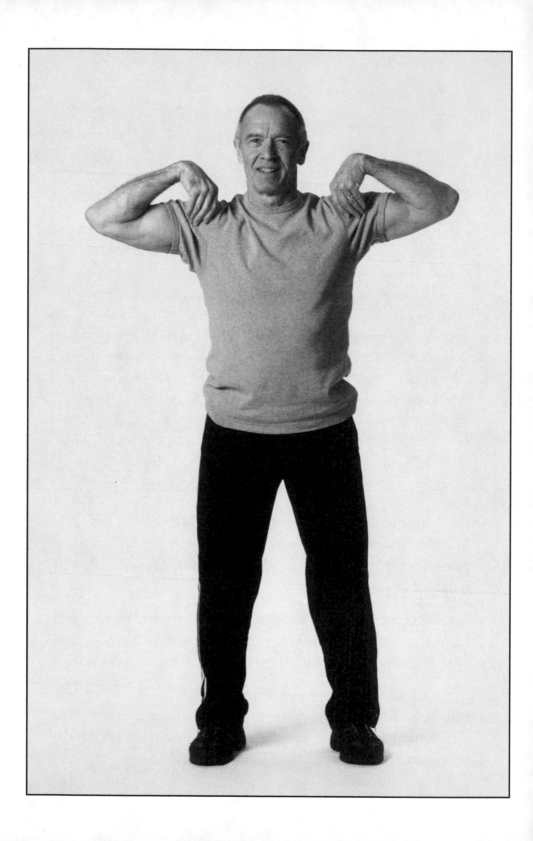

7

Range of Motion Exercises

As discussed in the last chapter, the goal of range of motion (ROM) exercises is to preserve joint function. Those kinds of exercises are helpful for those suffering from arthritis because they encourage you to move your limbs, head, neck, shoulders, torso, and feet, allowing the involved joint and surrounding structures to move more freely. In this chapter are ROM exercises that you can perform first thing in the morning and also during the rest of the day.

Performing ROM exercises upon wakening—even before getting out of bed—will get your blood circulating and ease morning stiffness. I suggest performing ROM exercises on a daily basis. They're low-level exercises that are easily tolerated.

Range of Motion Exercises

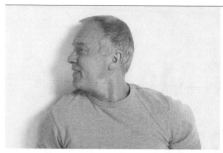

Neck Rolls, page 80

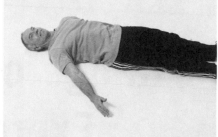

Shoulder Slide, page 81

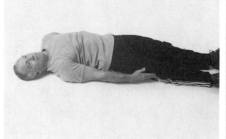

Mini Side Bend, page 82

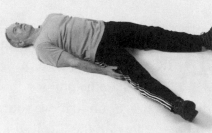

Hip Slide, page 83

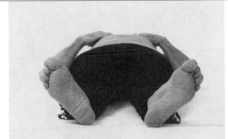

Hip Rotation, page 84

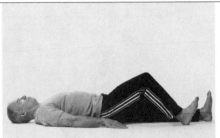

Hip & Knee Slide, page 85

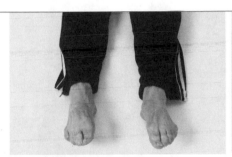

Ankle Flex , page 86

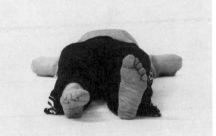

Ankle Circles, page 87

Range of Motion Exercises

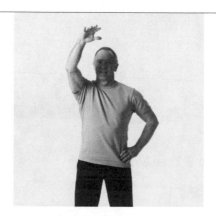

Single Arm Swoop, page 92

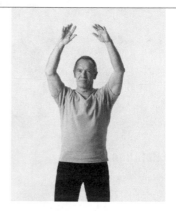

Double Arm Swoop, page 94

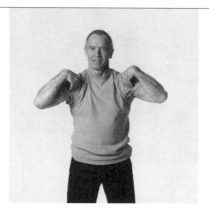

Shoulder Circles, page 96

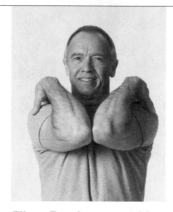

Elbow Touches, page 98

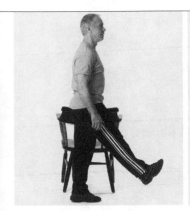

Leg Swings, page 100

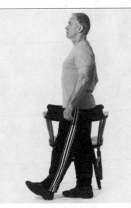

Knee Lifts, page 102

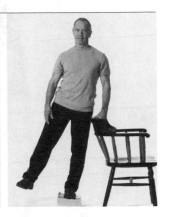

Side Leg Lifts, page 104

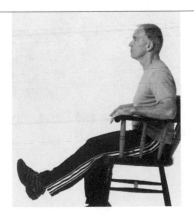

Seated Kicks, page 106

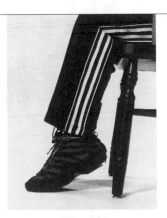

Calf Raises, page 108

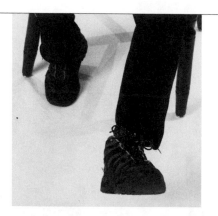

Ankle Circles, page 110

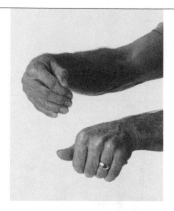

Wrist Circles, page 112

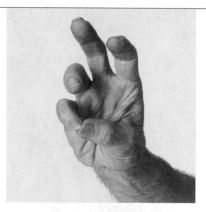

Finger Touches, page 114

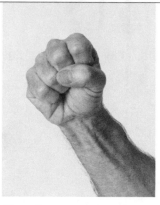

Fists Open and Close, page 115

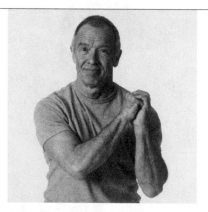

Chopping Wood, page 116

Morning Wake-Up Exercises to Start Your Day

Before you get out of bed, try these gentle, joint loosening exercises. Perform each exercise slowly and smoothly. Stay within your comfort zone. Never exceed your flexibility range. Remember, the purpose of these exercises is to gradually wake up your muscles and loosen your joints. Are you ready? Here are some pointers to keep in mind as you perform the exercises in this section.

* For each exercise, lie flat on your back and relax your body. Take a few deep breaths to oxygenate your blood.

* You may place a pillow under your knees if you experience any back discomfort. The fact that your body is fully supported, as you lie in your nice, warm, comfortable bed makes these exercises ideal for relieving morning stiffness.

* Perform 3 to 8 repetitions of each exercise, or as physical comfort allows.

Neck Rolls

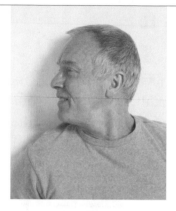

This exercise is very important since you use this movement when you drive your car—and you definitely want to maintain this range of motion to see cars behind you.

1 Start with your head centered, and look up toward the ceiling.

2 Rotate your head slowly to the right, looking over your right shoulder.

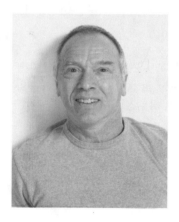

3 Slowly return to the center position. Repeat moving your head toward your left shoulder. Alternate moving your head to right–center–left–center.

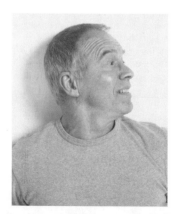

Shoulder Slide

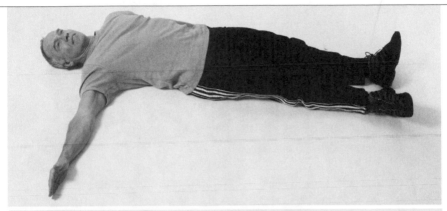

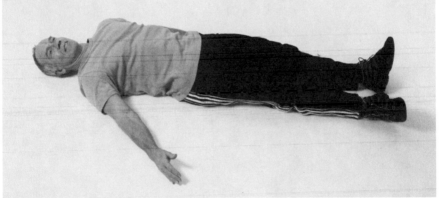

1. Lie so that your head and body are centered and your arms are relaxed at your sides, next to your body.

2. Raise your right arm slowly to the side, away from your body.

3. Return your arm to the starting position.

4. Repeat the movement with the left arm. Alternate the right and left arms.

Mini Side Bend

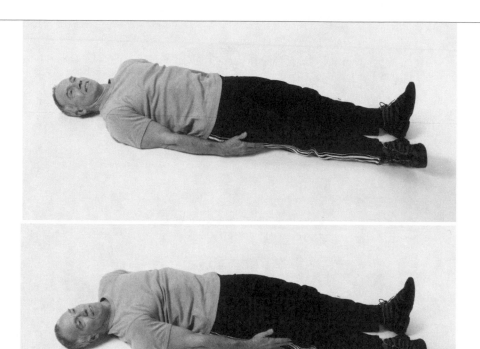

The bending action should come from the spine and waist—not the neck. Always keep your head, shoulders, and back in contact with the bed.

Note: If you have osteoporosis of the spine, consult your doctor before performing this exercise, since it may be contraindicated.

1. Start in the centered position.
2. Slowly bend to the right from your waist.
3. Reach your right hand toward your ankles.
4. Return to center. Repeat on the left side.

Hip Slide

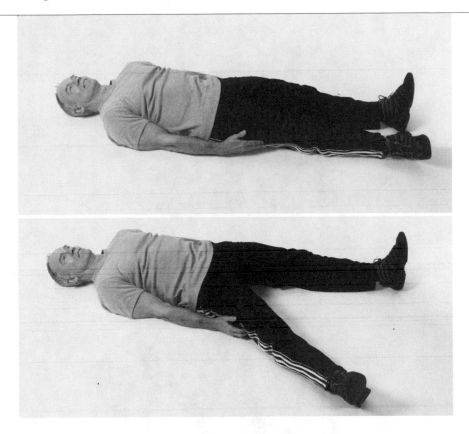

This exercise is similar to the Shoulder Slide, but you're using your legs instead. Make sure to keep your toes pointed toward the ceiling as you move your leg to the side.

1 Start with your body centered, relaxed and your legs together.

2 From this starting position, slowly slide your right leg out to the side, away from your body.

3 Slowly return the leg to center. Alternate the right and left legs.

Hip Rotation

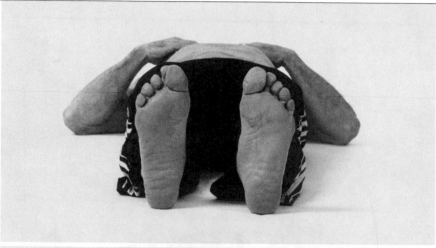

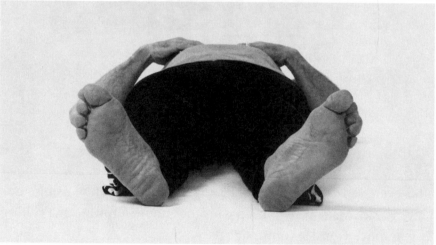

1. Lie with your feet 5 to 7 inches apart and your toes pointed toward the ceiling.

2. Rotate your hips outward so your feet point outward in a **V** shape.

3. Roll your feet back inward to the starting position.

Hip & Knee Slide

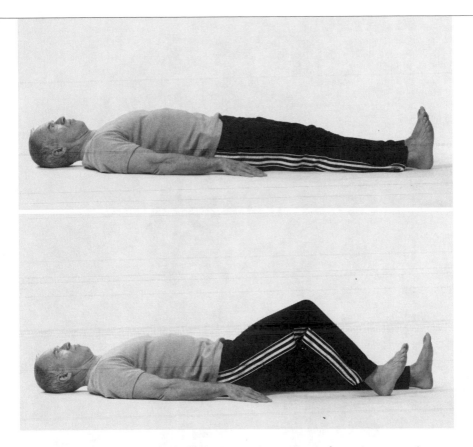

Remember for this—and all the morning range of motion exercises—to keep the body part you're moving in contact with the bed.

1 Start with your legs flat in the centered position.

2 Slide your right heel up and toward your right hips, bending your knee to approximately 90 degrees or within your comfort range. Keep your heel in contact with the bed.

3 Slowly straighten the right knee and repeat on the left leg. Alternate right and left legs.

Ankle Flex

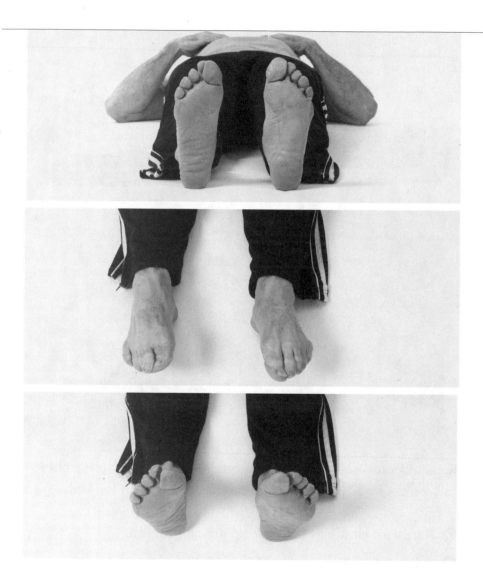

① Flex your foot, bringing your toes toward your shins.

② Return your foot to the starting position and then point your toes. Continue to move slowly between flexing and pointing.

Ankle Circles

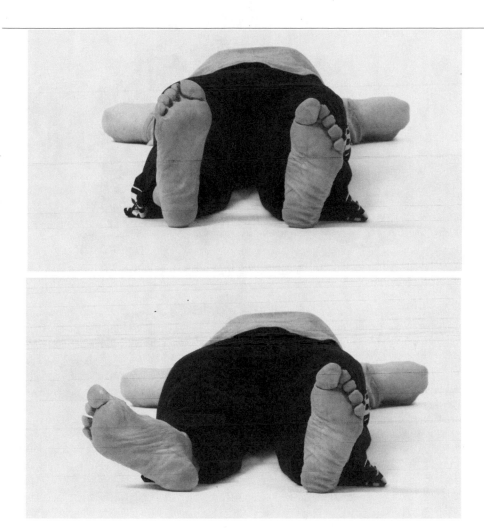

1. Slowly circle your right ankle in a clockwise motion.

2. Reverse direction and rotate the ankle in a counterclockwise direction.

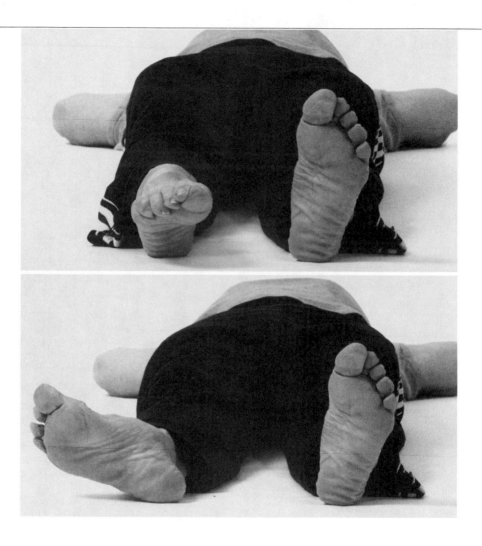

3 Repeat circles on the left foot, first moving in a clockwise and then counterclockwise direction.

Range of Motion Exercises for the Rest of the Day

The following exercises are designed to help you move your joints through their natural range of motion. You may not realize it, but often when you have pain and stiffness, you tend to limit your movements or try not to move your limbs at all. Over time, not fully extending or moving your joints will cause the muscles that serve the joint to become shortened (contracted) and weak.

+ Perform each exercise at a slow to moderate speed.

+ Movements should be well controlled. Again, stay within a comfort range of motion.

+ Each movement is followed by a stretch that complements the exercise and provides a period of rest.

+ Perform 3 to 8 repetitions of each exercise (or as tolerated) and hold each stretch for 20 seconds.

Before you get started turn on your favorite music to help you get motivated to move!

Posture

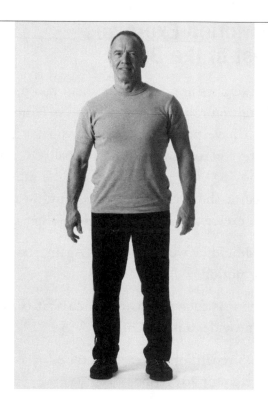

Remember what your mother told you to "stand up straight"? It's especially important for people with arthritis. Standing with poor posture places an unnecessary burden on your already vulnerable joints. Establish a good foundation before you start exercising—stand tall. Here's how:

❶ Stack the head, neck and spine like a column. The head and neck should flow directly up out of your spine.

❷ The tips of your shoulders should point out to the sides. Try to create an equal relationship or distance between the sternum and the shoulders and the spine and the shoulders. In other

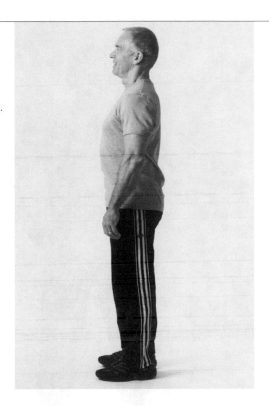

words, their should be an equal pull on the shoulders from the front and the back.

3 Have someone check your postural alignment from the side. Your ear lobes should be directly in line with the tips of your shoulders. Your shoulders should be in line with your hips and ankles. Maintaining proper posture during exercise will mini-mize muscle strain.

Single Arm Swoop

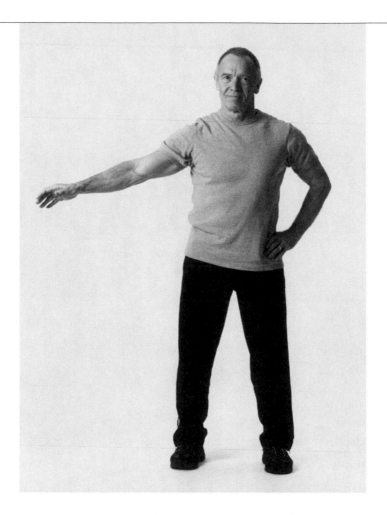

1. Stand with your feet shoulder-width apart. Do not lock your knees.

2. Place your left hand on your left hip.

3. Start with your right arm down, at your side.

4. Swoop the right arm in an arc up, over, and slightly in front of your head.

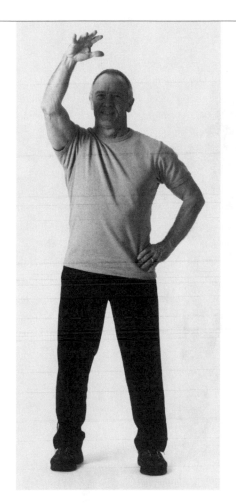 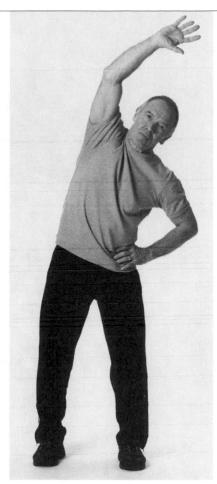

⑤ In a single fluid motion, bring it down following the same arc. Now for the stretch.

⑥ On the last repetition, keep the arm up and hold the stretch. You should feel a lengthening through the torso, upper back and your arm. You can bend slightly to the side to increase the stretch. Keep your opposite arm on your hip to help support your back. Repeat with the left arm.

Double Arm Swoop

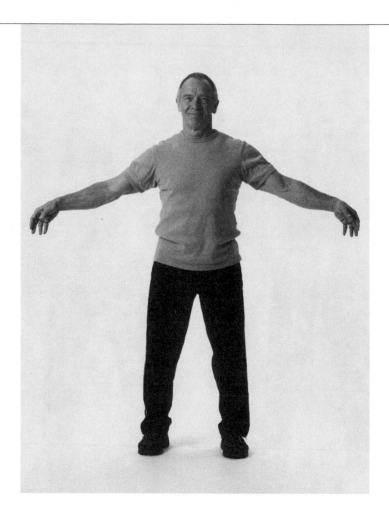

This exercise is similar to the Single Arm Swoop, except that both arms are used.

1 Stand with your feet shoulder-width apart. Do not lock your knees.

2 Place your hands on your hips.

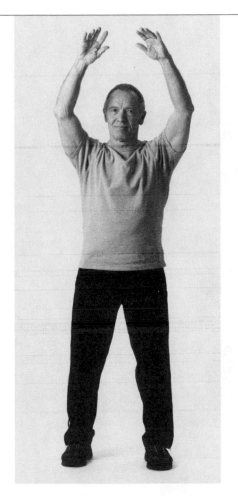 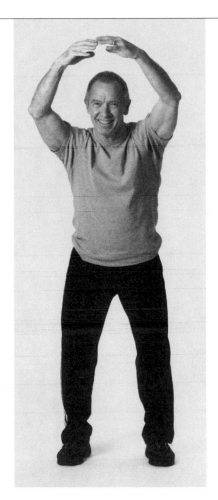

3 Swoop both arms up and then lower them.

4 Hold the stretch with both arms up, hands clasped, and slightly in front of the head.

Shoulder Circles

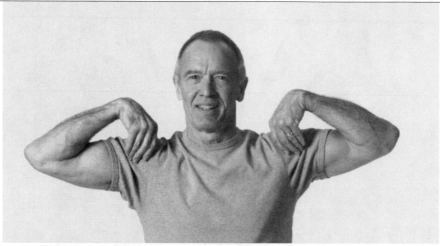

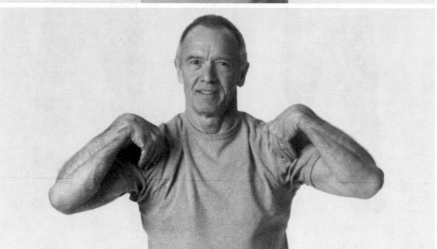

❶ Place your hands on your shoulders and raise your elbows to the sides.

❷ Imagine the points of your elbow are pencils, and draw clockwise circles with them. Start out doing small circles and gradually, as the joint becomes looser, draw larger circles. Continue drawing circles.

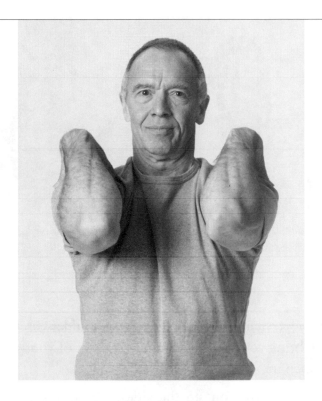

③ Gradually begin moving your elbows to the front at chest level, while continuing to draw the circles.

④ For the stretch, touch the elbows together (see page 98), or bring them close together, and hold the position. You should feel the stretch in your upper back, throughout the shoulder blades.

⑤ Repeat the exercise, this time making circles in a counter-clockwise direction.

Elbow Touches

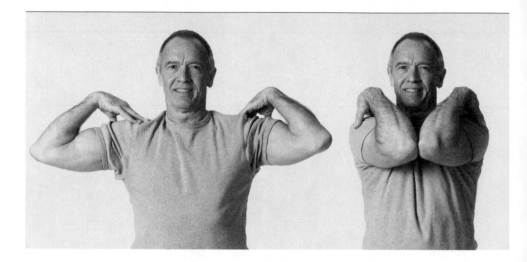

1. From the stretch position in Step 4 of Shoulder Circles (previous page), bring your elbows together in front of your chest and then open up the chest

2. Bring the elbows out to the sides. Slowly repeat the motion touching the elbows to the front and bringing them out to the sides.

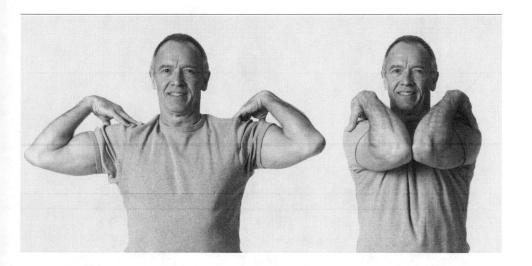

3 For the stretch, maintaining the same positioning of the arms, press your elbows to the back. Feel your chest open and expand. You should also feel a stretch through the front of the shoulders.

Leg Swings

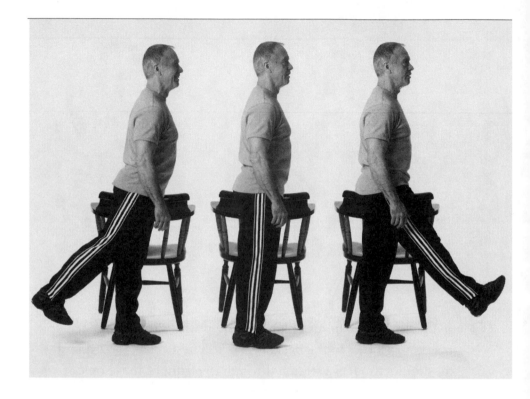

① Stand (with good posture) with the side of your body to the back of a chair.

② Using the back of the chair for support, lift the outside leg to the chair to the front.

③ With a smooth, controlled motion, bring your leg to the back. Keep your back straight, your abdominal muscles contracted, and the knee of the supporting leg slightly bent.

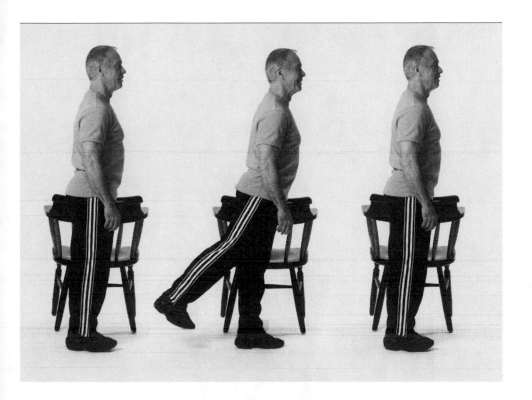

④ Continue the motion, swinging the leg to the front and back. You may pause in the center position if it is more comfortable to do so.

⑤ Turn and face the opposite direction and repeat on the opposite leg.

Knee Lifts

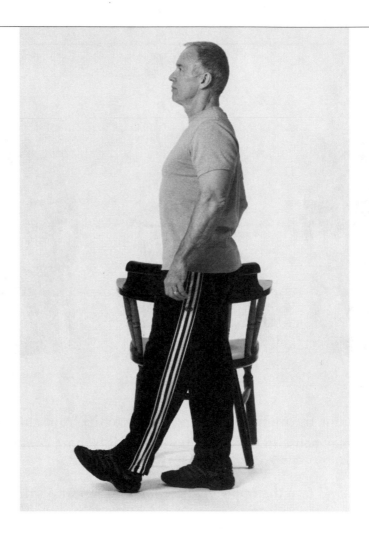

As you perform this exercise, make sure not to lift the knee higher than the hip.

1 Stand (with good posture) with the side of your body to the back of a chair.

2 Lift your knee to the front.

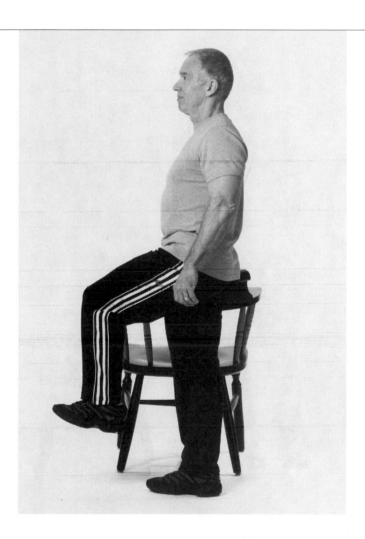

3 Lower your leg back to the floor. Continue to lift and lower the knee.

Side Leg Lifts

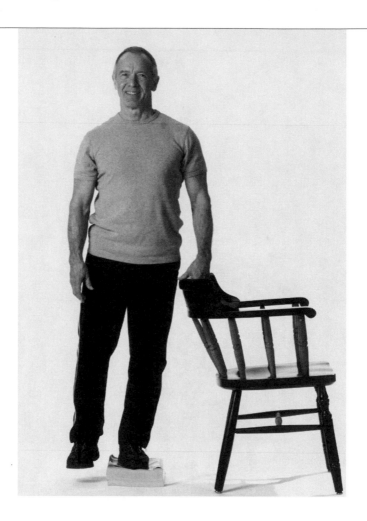

As you do this exercise, keep your back and hips straight. Don't lean to the side in order to lift your leg higher. Finally, the height of the lift should be within your comfort range.

① Stand with your left side to the back of a chair and your left foot on top of a block or thick phone book. Keep your body

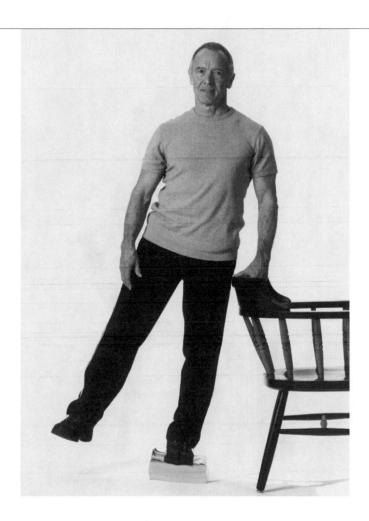

weight distributed evenly over both feet, even though one foot is not being supported. Hold the chair with your left hand.

2 Lift your right leg out to the side and then return to the starting position. Alternate right and left leg lifts to the side.

Seated Kicks

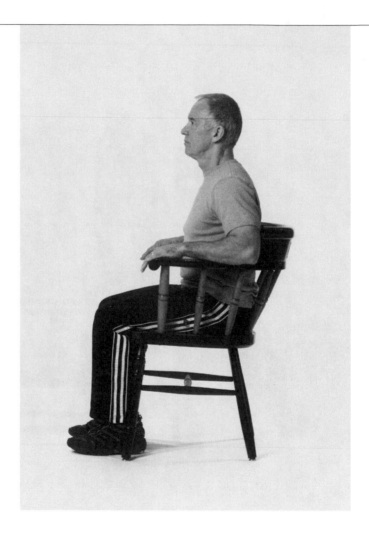

1 Sit in a chair with your back fully supported. Your feet should be flat on the floor and positioned under your knees.

2 Straighten the right knee, kicking the leg to the front.

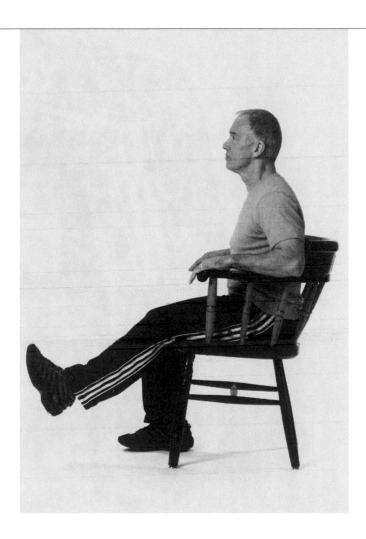

It is not necessary to fully extend the leg if it is uncomfortable. Keep your upper thigh in contact with the seat of the chair as you alternate lifting and lowering the right and left legs.

Calf Raises

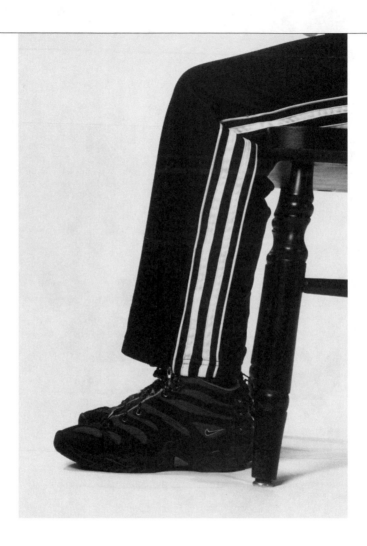

➊ Sit straight but comfortably in a chair with your feet flat on the floor.

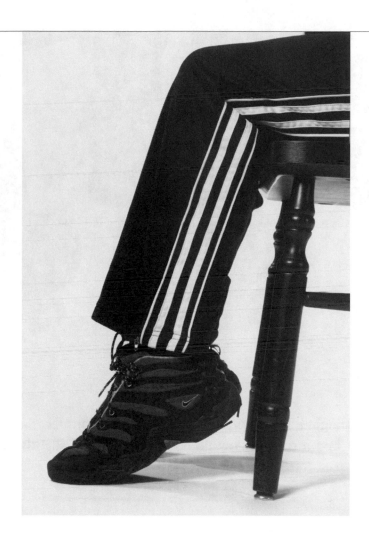

2 Lift and lower your heels either one at a time or both together.

Ankle Circles

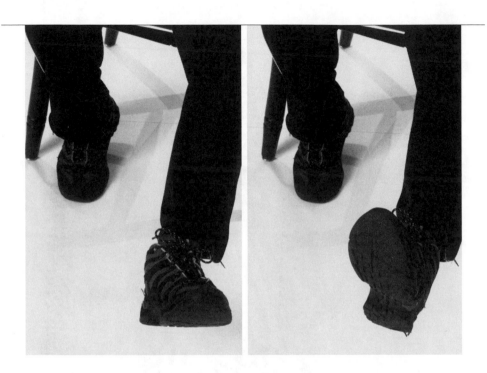

1 Sit straight but comfortably in a chair with your feet flat on the floor and a small pillow under your thighs to slightly elevate your legs.

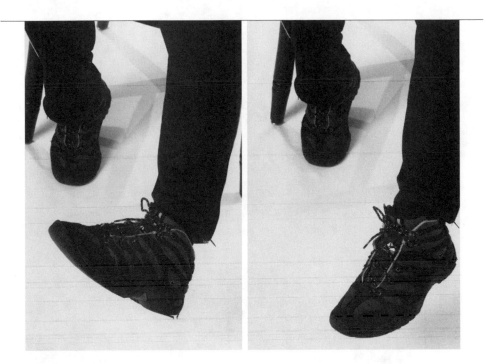

2 Circle the right ankle clockwise and then counterclockwise.

3 Repeat with the left ankle.

Wrist Circles

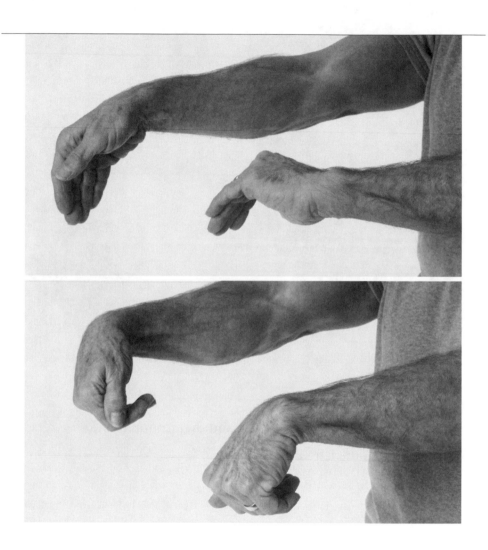

Circle the wrists in clockwise and counterclockwise directions.

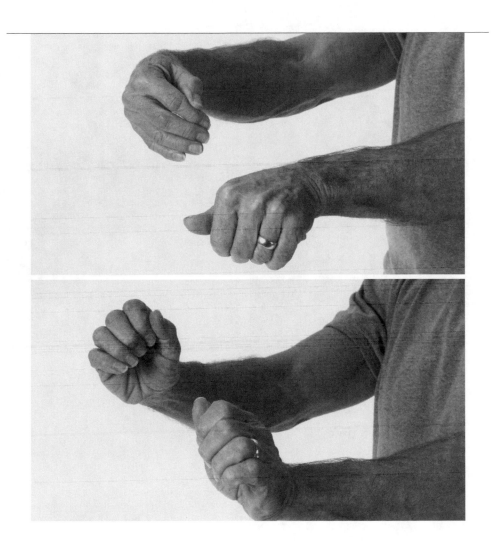

Finger Touches

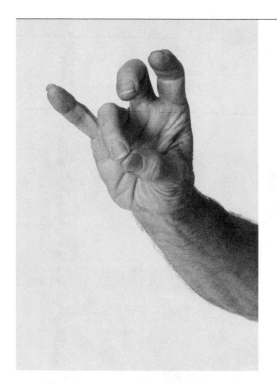 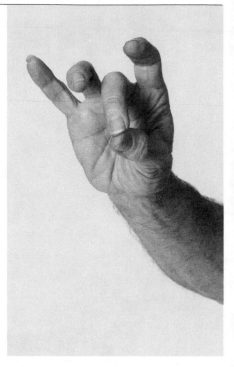

1 Touch each finger to the thumb.

2 Repeat 3 to 5 times

Fists Open and Close

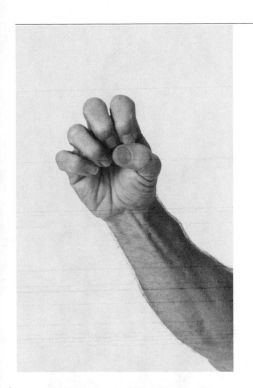 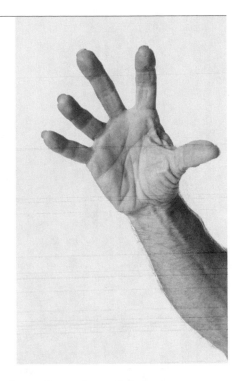

1 Close your hands in a fist but don't squeeze them tight.

2 Slowly open your hands and spread your fingers.

3 Repeat 3 to 5 times.

Chopping Wood

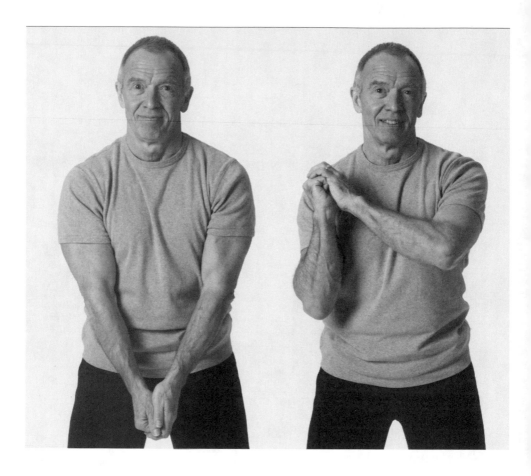

1. Stand with your arms at your sides.

2. Clasp your hands together and hold your arms are held straight down.

3. Bend your elbows and bring both hands up to the right shoulder.

4. Return to the starting position.

5. Bend the elbows again and bring the hands up to the left shoulder.

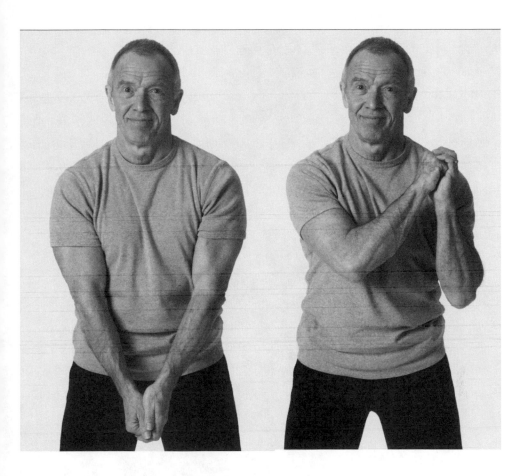

6 Continue the exercise, alternating the chopping motion to the right and left shoulders.

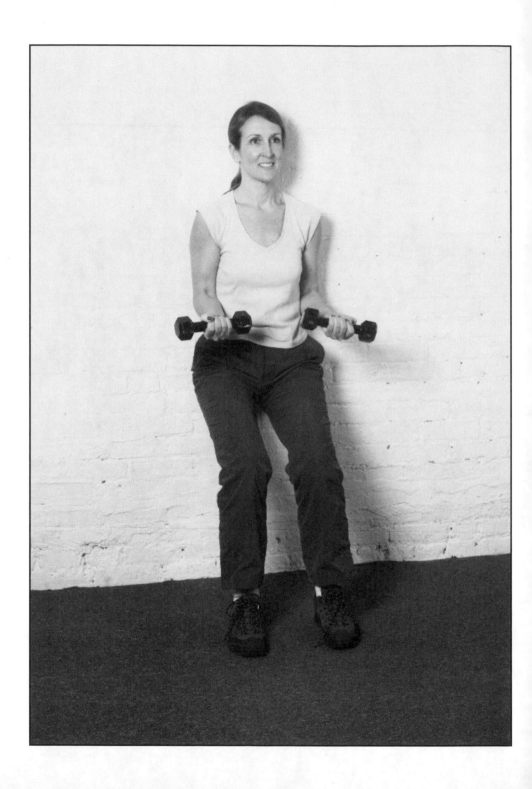

8

Isometric Exercises for Strength Training

When your muscle contracts it shortens. This type of contraction is called *isotonic*. Muscle contraction is said to be *isometric* when the muscle does not shorten during contraction.

Strength training, using isometric contractions, is ideal for your arthritis because it is performed without movement. Brief isometric (held) contractions will strengthen the muscle without involving the joint. Here's how to perform the exercises in this section.

+ Perform each exercise 1 to 8 times.
+ Hold each position for 3 to 6 seconds.
+ Rest for 20 seconds between each contraction.
+ Perform these exercises with or without weights. I suggest using 1- to 3-pound hand weights, as tolerated

Isometric Exercises for Strength Training

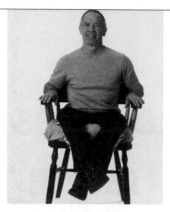

Seated Cross-Legged Press,
page 124

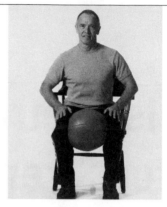

Seated Inner Thigh Squeeze,
page 125

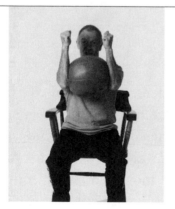

Seated Chest Press, page 126

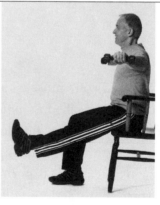

Seated Airplanes, page 127

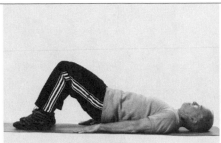

Pelvic Tilt, page 128

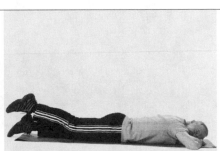

Prone Leg Lift, page 129

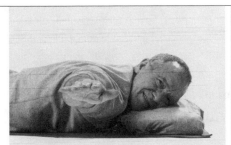

Prone Arm Lift, page 130

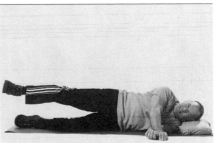

Side Leg Lifts, page 131

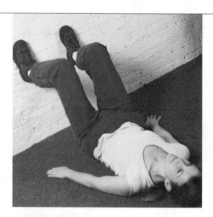

Wall Press, page 132

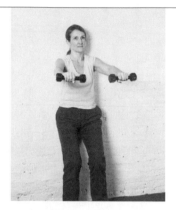

Wall Sitting, or Elevator Up, Elevator Down, page 133

Other Strength-Training Exercises

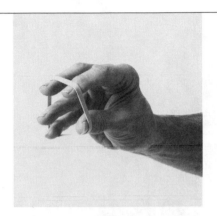

Rubber Band Stretch, page 137

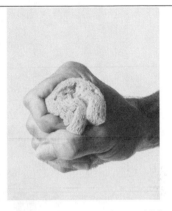

Sponge Squeeze, page 138

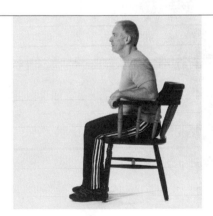

Sit to Stand, page 139

Seated Cross-Legged Press

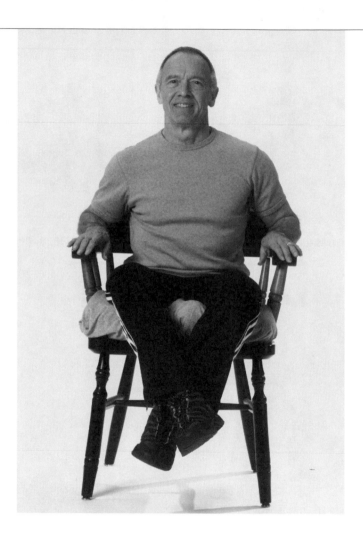

1. Sit on a chair with a pillow under your knees.
2. Cross the right ankle over the left ankle.
3. Press the right leg against the left leg. At the same time, press the left leg forward against the right.
4. Hold the press for 3 to 6 seconds and release.
5. Change position and place the left leg over the right. Repeat.

Seated Inner Thigh Squeeze

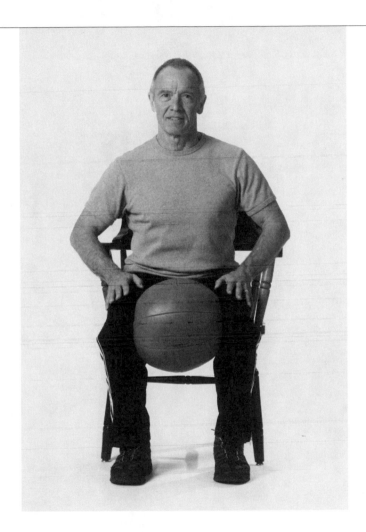

For this you can use any type of ball you have around: the kids' kickball, a basketball or soccer ball, or even a small medicine ball.

1. Sit on a chair with a ball between your legs.

2. Gently squeeze the ball with your thighs. Hold the position for 3 to 6 seconds and then release.

Seated Chest Press

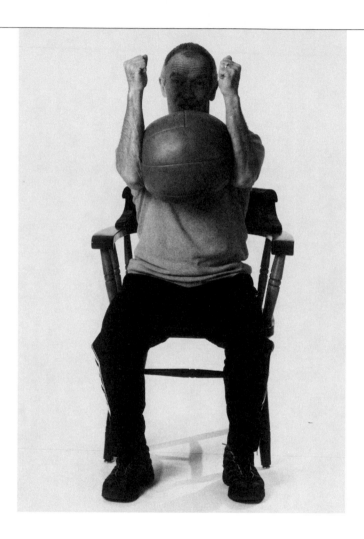

1. Sit on a chair, holding a ball in front of you between your elbows.

2. Squeeze the ball.

3. Hold the squeeze for 3 to 6 seconds, while taking deep, slow breaths.

4. Release and repeat.

Seated Airplanes

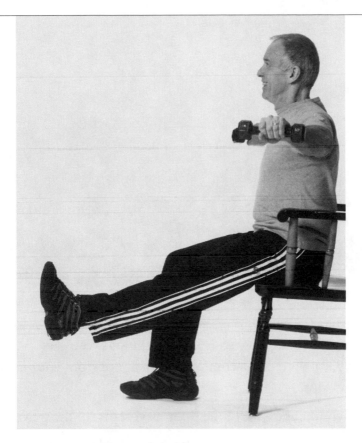

When you raise your arms while doing this exercise, do not lift them higher than your shoulders. As your strength increases, start using light (1- to 3-pound) hand weights.

1. Sit on a chair with a pillow behind your back for support.

2. Lift one leg straight out in front of you and lift both arms to the sides As you hold the position, keep your back straight and your abdominal muscles pulled in.

3. Repeat the exercise by lifting the opposite leg and raising your arms out in front of you.

Pelvic Tilt

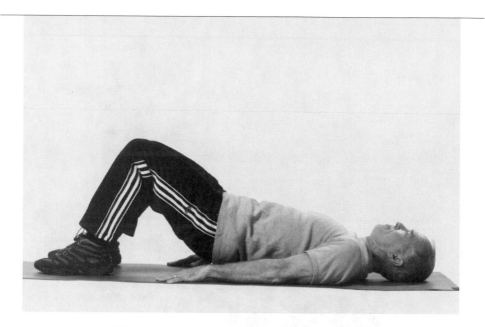

1. Lie on your back with your knees bent and your feet flat on the floor. Keep your feet a comfortable distance from your hips, but not too close.

2. Press your spine toward the floor as you tilt up the pelvis.

3. Lift your tailbone and lower back off the floor, but keep your mid- and upper back in contact with the floor. You should feel the contraction in your buttock and abdomen. Hold the position while taking slow, deep breaths.

Prone Leg Lift

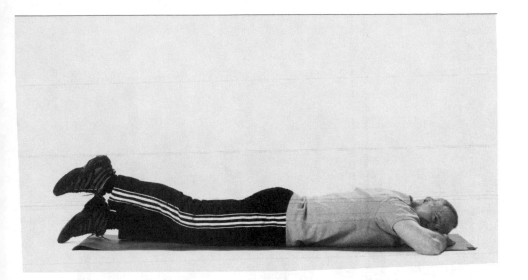

❶ Lie face down on the floor.

❷ Lift one leg a few inches from the floor and hold the contraction. During this lift the hips should remain in contact with the floor.

Prone Arm Lift

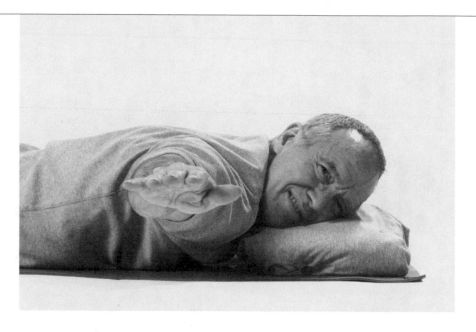

1 Lie face down on the floor.

2 Bring your arms out to the sides. Lift the arms a few inches from the floor and hold the contraction.

Side Leg Lifts

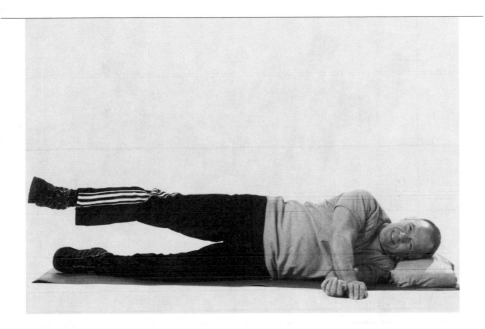

This is a great exercise to strengthen your hip and outer thigh muscles.

1 Lie on your side, using a pillow to support your head.

2 Extend your top leg out to the side and bend the bottom leg slightly in front of you.

3 Lift your top leg to approximately hip height and hold the position.

Wall Press

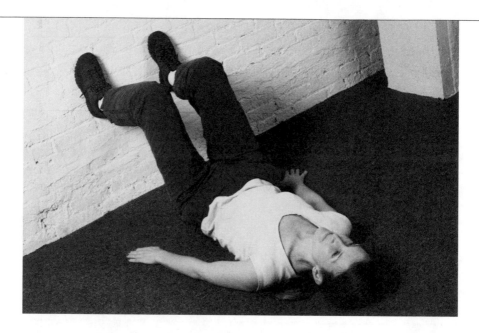

As you press during this exercise, you may tighten your abdominal muscles and lift your shoulders slightly.

1. Lie flat on your back with your knees bent at a 90-degree angle and your feet flat against a wall.

2. Gently press your feet into the wall. You should feel the tension in your buttocks and thigh muscles.

3. Hold the position for 3 to 6 seconds, and then release.

Wall Sitting, *or* Elevator Up, Elevator Down

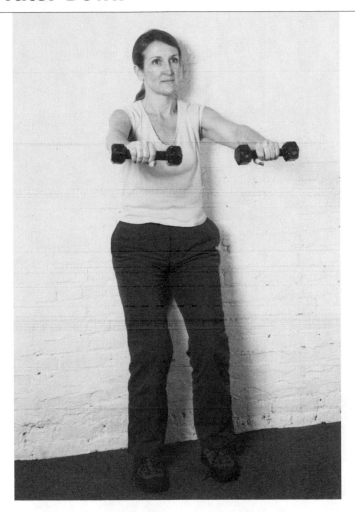

When you do this exercise, you need to have your feet far enough away from the wall so as you bend your knees, they stay behind the toes. You may use 1- to 3-pound weights as you do this exercise.

1 Stand with your back, shoulders, and head flat against a wall. Step your feet 1 to 1 1/2 feet in front of you.

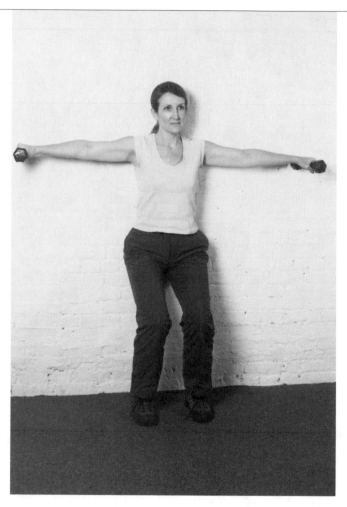

2 Bend your knees, raise your arms in front of you, and drop your hips approximately 3 inches. Hold this position for 3 to 8 seconds, keeping your abdominal muscles held in.

3 Drop down another 3 inches and move your arms to your sides.

4 If you're able, bend your knees and lower your body another 3 inches. Hold the arms in a biceps curl position.

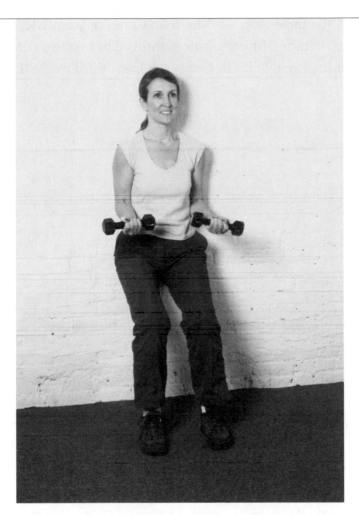

⑤ Now reverse the exercise, raising yourself 3 inches, holding the position, raising yourself another 3 inches, holding the position, and finally, returning to the start position.

⑥ As you return to the start position, slowly uncurl your arms, returning them to the starting position.

Other Strength-Training Exercises

Although the three exercises that follow are not isometric, they are still useful for those suffering from arthritis. The first two concentrate on increasing strength in the hands, while the third works the legs.

Rubber Band Stretch

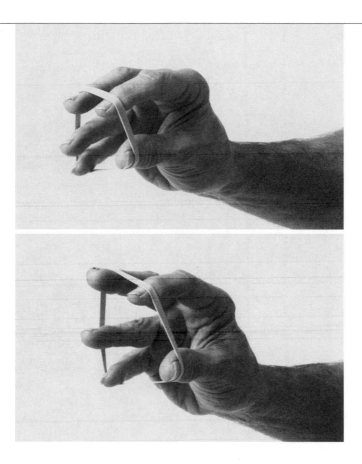

① Place a rubber band around all five fingers so that it lays between the base of the fingernail and the first joint.

② Spread your fingers apart from each other as far as you can. Slowly release the tension of the rubber band, returning your hand to its starting position.

Sponge Squeeze

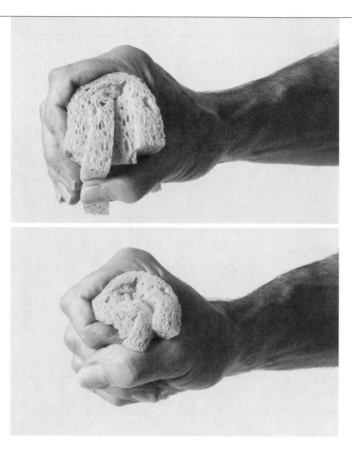

1 Dampen a medium household sponge.

2 Holding the sponge in one hand, squeeze and release the sponge. Repeat 8 to 10 times.

3 Repeat with the opposite hand.

Sit to Stand

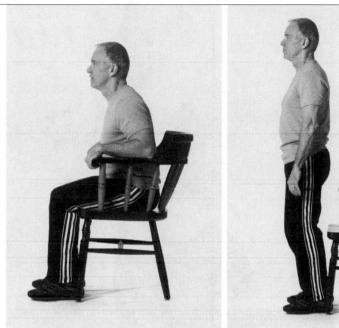 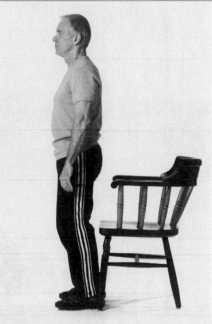

The Sit to Stand is a great exercise to strengthen your legs. Use a high seated chair with arm rests.

1. Sit on the chair with your arms on the arm rests and your feet directly under your knees.

2. Slowly rise to a standing position and then slowly lower yourself to the seated position. Repeat.

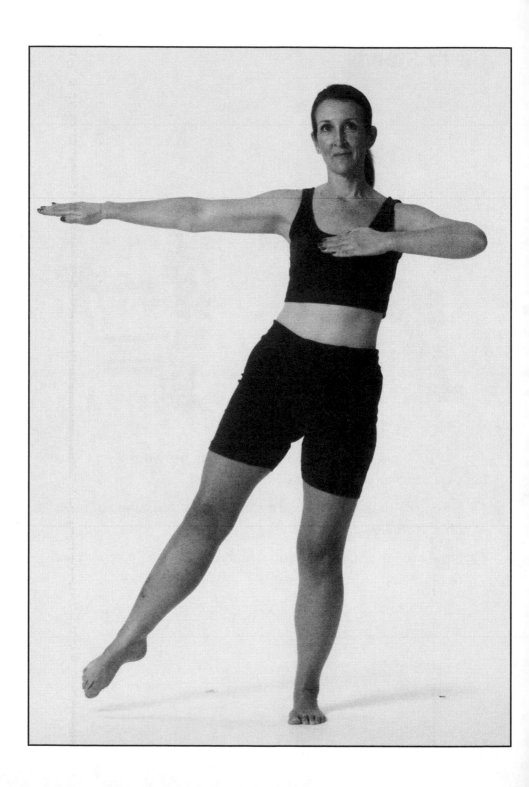

9

Cardiovascular Training for Arthritis

Cardiovascular Conditioning

Cardiovascular conditioning, also called aerobic conditioning, involves rhythmically moving large muscle groups (such as the big muscles in the legs), at the right intensity and continuously, for at least 20 to 30 minutes. Moving large muscles is necessary to increase the blood flow (and therefore oxygen) throughout the body and back to the heart. It is that increase in blood flow that strengthens the heart, making it a more effective and healthier pumping muscle. Examples of cardiovascular conditioning activities include walking, running, swimming, aerobics, and biking. All are good ways to increase your aerobic fitness.

The American College of Sports Medicine has issued the following guidelines for healthy aerobic activity:

- Exercise 3 to 5 days of each week.

- Warm up for 5 to 10 minutes before starting the aerobic activity.

- Maintain your exercise intensity for 30 to 45 minutes and then gradually decrease the intensity of your work out before cooling down.

Starting a Walking Program

There's a difference between walking for locomotion (to get from one point to another) and walking to develop physical fitness. When walking for fitness, you must pay attention to form, technique, walking pace, and attire.

A moderate to brisk walking pace—3 to 4.5 miles per hour (mph) or at a 13- to 19-minute per mile pace—is an excellent goal to work toward. Appropriate exercise progression is important both to prevent injury and to help you stick to the program. If you fatigue easily, start slowly and then gradually pick up the pace. You may want to start out walking on your local high school track. Typically, those tracks are a quarter-mile long. If you walk around one four times (for a total of one mile) and time how long it takes, you'll get an idea of your walking pace. Once you get the "feel" for an appropriate pace, which should be fairly light to somewhat difficult, then begin to walk throughout your neighborhood or park. Walking faster or walking up hills can increase the intensity of your walks. Vary the walking route to include hills or more different terrain such as sand.

Technique

The most important aspect of effective walking technique is alignment. Good posture is the foundation of efficient and safe fitness walking. Your head should be held in a neutral, centered position, in line with your spine. Your chin should be parallel to the ground. Keep your focus to the front. Your shoulders are held down, back, and relaxed. This allows your arms to swing with a greater range of motion. Your chest should be lifted and expanded to facilitate breathing. Your abdominal muscles should be held in gently. Additionally, your buttocks should be tucked under your hips, maintaining proper alignment of the spine.

Swing your arms from the shoulder joint and close to the sides of your body. Your arms should follow a direct line from the back to the front. Avoid swinging them side to side like windshield wipers. Swing your arms no higher than the shoulders. As your speed increases, bend your elbows approximately 90 degrees. Use a pumping action to increase the intensity. Your hands should be held in a loose fist. Keep the wrists straight.

Leg Action

Stride length should be comfortable, but varies among individuals. The length of your stride is determined by your leg length and hamstring flexibility. Try to produce a smooth and fluid action, the hip come forward as you step out with your foot. As your foot is placed on the ground, it should roll from heel to toe. Avoid pounding the foot down. Push off the forefoot at the completion of each step. Lean forward from the ankle, not the hip, to increase speed. This will reduce stress to the back.

Apparel

If you plan to make walking a regular part of your exercise program, then it is important to purchase appropriate sneakers. The heel should provide good support and the forefoot should be flexible. Dress in layers so that you can remove clothing as you warm up. During hot weather, exercise during the cool part of the day and decrease the intensity of your exercise. Heart rate tends to run higher during exercise in hot or humid weather.

Water Exercises for Cardiovascular Training

When I suggest exercising in the water some people respond, "but I don't know how to swim," or, "I'm not a good swimmer." Let me assure you that being a good swimmer is not necessary to get the benefits of exercise in the water. The exercises designed for this book are performed in the shallow end of a pool.

Water's elements—buoyancy, turbulence, and resistance—make it an ideal environment for exercise. When your body is immersed in water you feel the buoyancy and massaging action created by the turbulence of the water as you move. The force or pressure of the water against your body provides support and reduces stress on the joints. When you perform these exercises you'll notice that the water provides resistance in both directions, through the full range of motion. Water exercise can therefore improve strength as well as cardiovascular fitness.

Before you start your water exercise program you need to follow a few guidelines.

1. The Arthritis Foundation recommends that the water temperature be between 83°F and 85°F, the ideal range for exercise. If the

water is too cold you'll be uncomfortable and become stiff and tense. Warm water causes your blood vessels to dilate, which in turn increases circulation. Increased circulation raises your muscles' temperature, allowing them to relax and move with ease.

2. Be aware of your body alignment. Always stand with good posture. Both feet should be flat on the level bottom of the pool. The water level should be at your lower ribs or nipples. Pull in your navel toward your spine. Keep your shoulders over your hips.

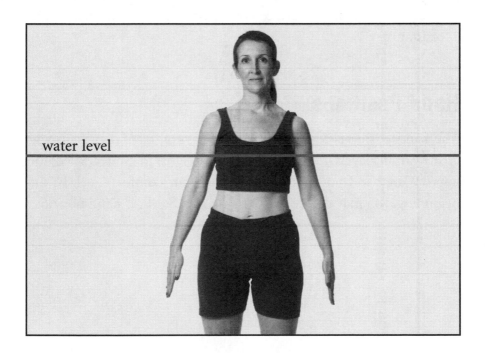

water level

3. Wear a form-fitting bathing suit to avoid excessive drag in the water. Aqua sneakers, which can be purchased at most sporting goods stores, will protect your feet.

4. There are several ways to control the intensity of water exercise:

   ◆ Increase or decrease the speed of your movement.

   ◆ Travel or move through the water to increase the intensity or exercise in place to decrease the intensity.

   ◆ Large movements are more intense than smaller movements, so adjust the range of motion according to your abilities or how you feel.

   ◆ Increase or decrease the drag forces during exercise. This relates to your body surface area as it moves and is resisted by the water. The greater the body surface area used will create an increase in resistance.

Hand Positions

The hand positions featured on the following pages can help you create varying levels of drag or resistance against the water. Select the appropriate hand position according to your comfort level. In the beginning, you may decide to use primarily the Slicer hand position.

Hand Positions

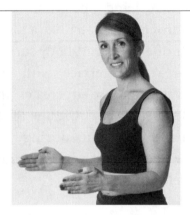

Slicer, page 148

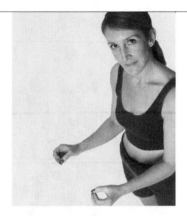

Donut, page 148

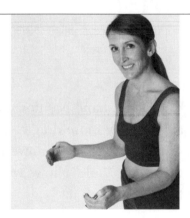

Cups, page 150

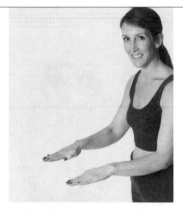

Flat Paddles, page 150

Slicer

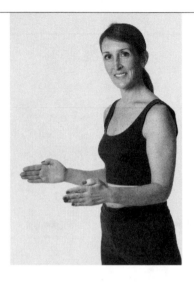

This hand position cuts through the water like a knife. It offers the least body surface area to interface with the water, and so it creates the least resistance. Use the Slicer hand position during the warm-up or if you find yourself getting tired.

Donut

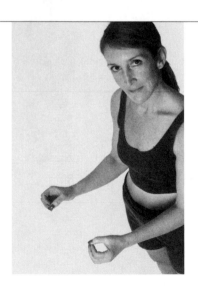

The Donut hand position creates slightly more drag in the water than the Slicer; however, the donut "hole" allows water to pass through it.

Cups

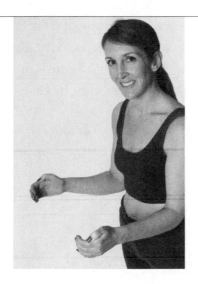

This hand position is the next step up in intensity. Cup your hands and pull them through the water. You will feel more resistance than with the Donut or Slicer.

Flat Paddles

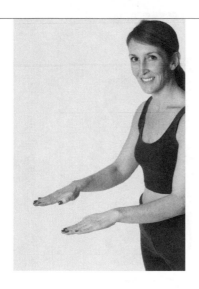

This hand position is similar to the Slicer but instead of slicing the water, you press the palm or back of the hand through the water. Flat Paddles provide the greatest resistance.

Upper Body Movements

The following upper body movements are presented in the order of difficulty or intensity. As with any exercise program, start at a low level of intensity to allow the body to adjust to the activity. To make the exercises easier, keep the movements small. If you want to make them more difficult increase the range of motion by making them larger.

Hand positions are given for each upper body movement.

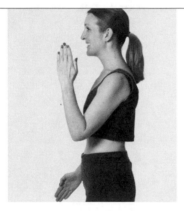

Arm Pumps, page 152

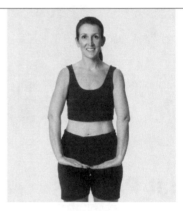

Presses, page 154

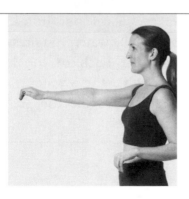

Reach and Rake, page 156

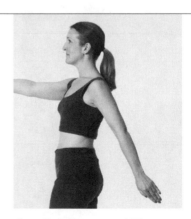

Arm Swings, page 158

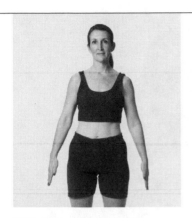

Side Raises, page 160

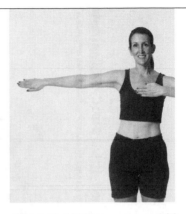

Windshield Wipers, page 162

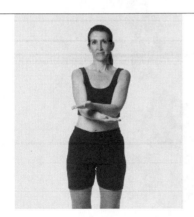

Figure 8s, page 164

Arm Pumps

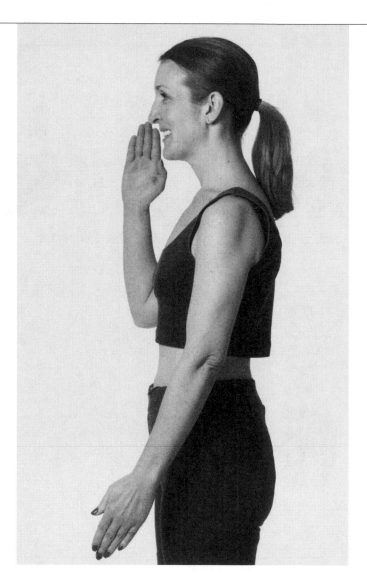

Keep with your elbows down at your sides. Bend and straighten your elbows in opposition to each other. As the right arm comes up, the left arm moves down.

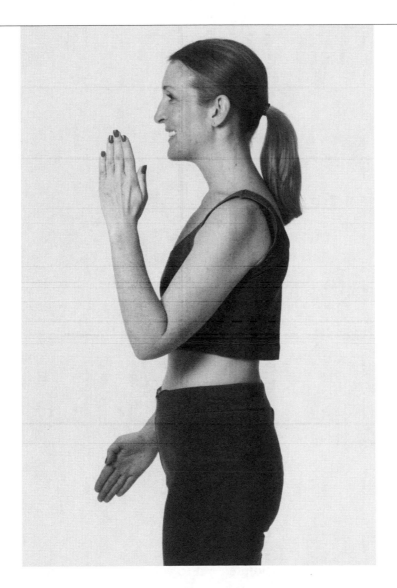

Hand positions: Slicer, Donut

Presses

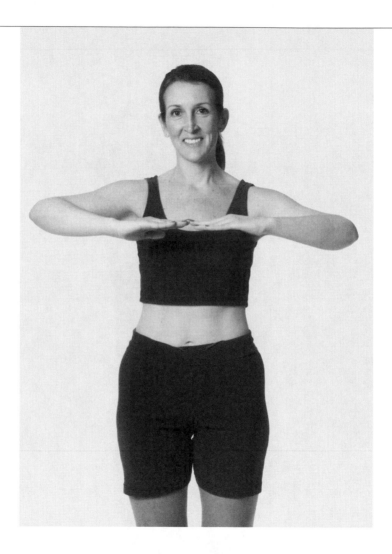

Start with your elbows pointed out to your sides. Your palms should be face down at chest level. Press your palms downward until the arms are almost fully extended. Return to the starting position.

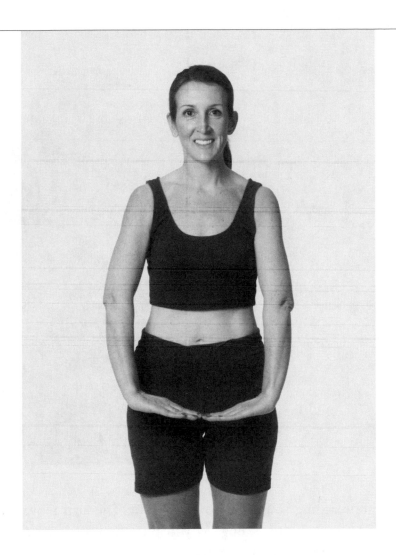

Hand position: Flat Paddles

Reach and Rake

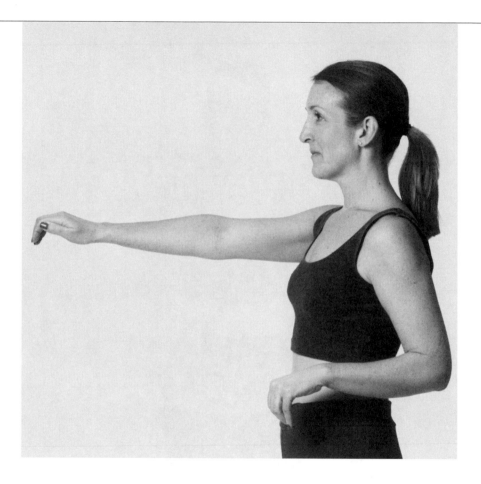

Alternate reaching your arms to your front. The arm movements resemble cross-country skiing. As you pull the water toward you, pretend you are raking the water.

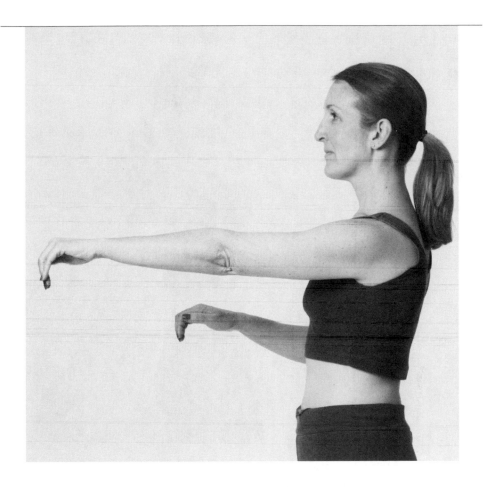

Hand position: Cups

Arm Swings

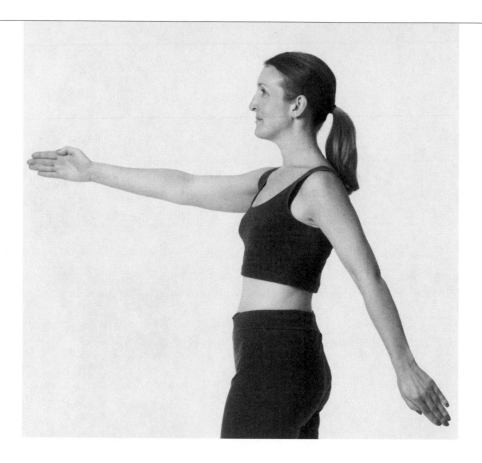

Start with your arms down at your sides. Scissor your arms front and back. Keep your elbows slightly bent. Try not to let the arms swing too far behind your hips. The movement here occurs from the shoulders, and not the elbows.

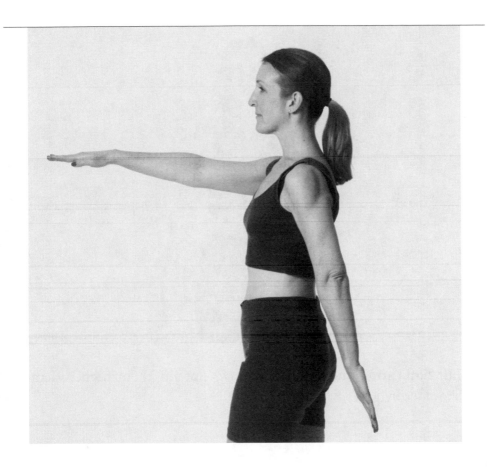

Hand positions: Start with the Slicer and Donut and progress to Flat Paddles.

Side Raises

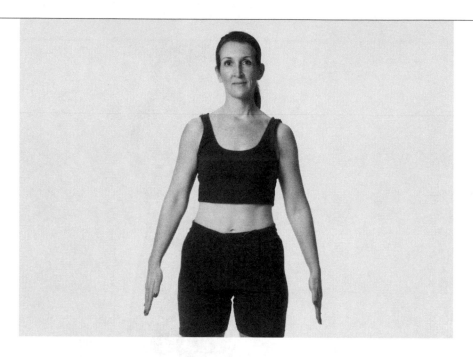

Lift both arms out to the sides. Do not lift them higher than shoulder height.

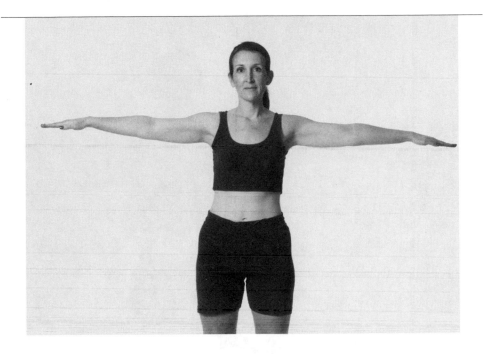

Hand position: Flat Paddles

Windshield Wipers

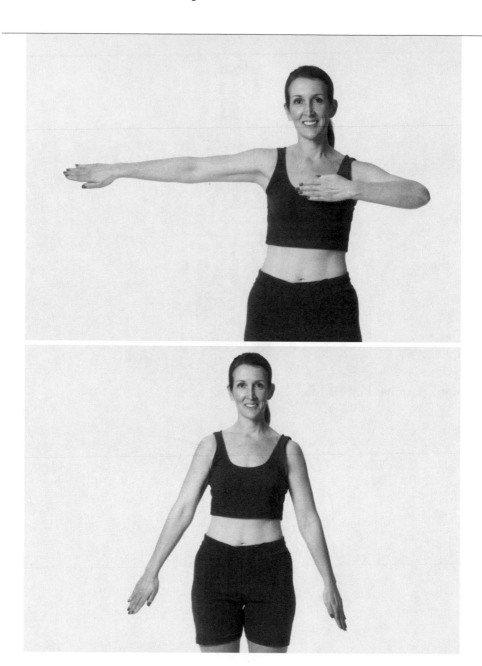

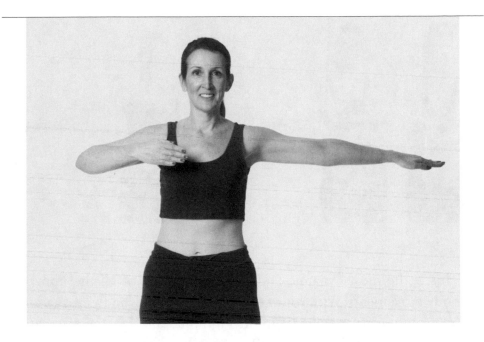

Swing both arms to the right and left, like windshield wipers. Your arms should travel in a path fairly close to the body. A variation of this exercise is to perform it at chest level, moving the arms on a horizontal plane.

Hand position: Slicer

Figure 8s

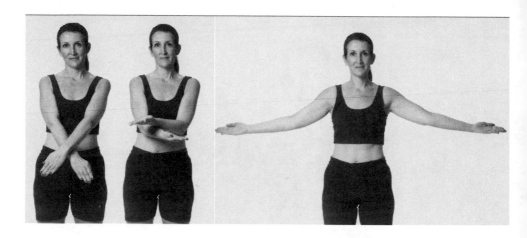

This is the most dynamic and fluid movement of all the upper body movements. With your arms in front of your body, cross and open your arms, moving them through the water in a figure-eight pattern. Start small and gradually increase the size of the eights. As you cross your arms to the front, your palms should face down. As you open your arms and bring them out to the sides, your palms should face up.

Lower Body Movements

The following lower body movements are presented in order of increasing intensity. The complementary upper body movements are given for each lower body movement. Use the hand positions that are given for the arm exercises.

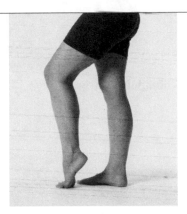

Prances, page 168

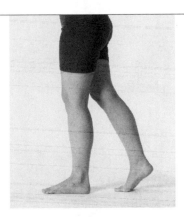

Water Walking, page 169

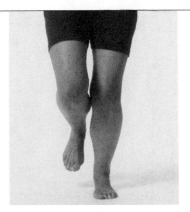

Water Jog, page 170

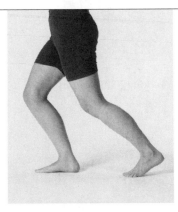

Scissors, page 171

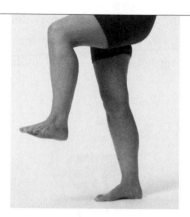

Knee Hops, page 172

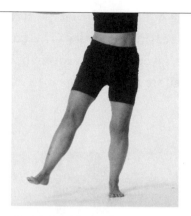

Pendulum Swings, page 173

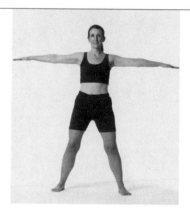

Jumping Jacks, page 174

Prances

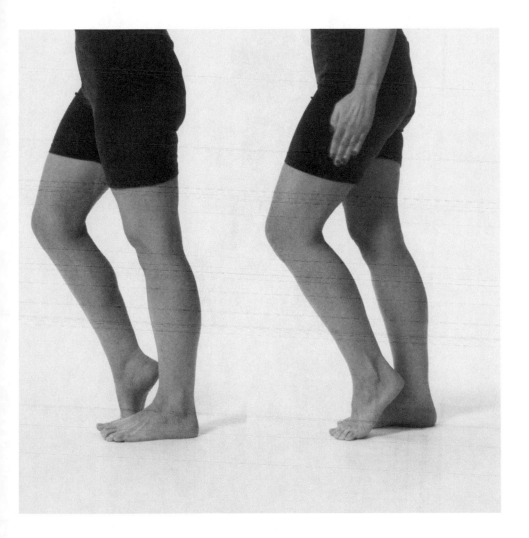

Begin with your feet shoulder width apart.

Alternate lifting your right and left heel. Keep the ball of the foot and toes in contact with the bottom of the pool. As you warm up, push off from the ball of the foot so your foot lifts slightly away from the pool bottom.

Upper body: Pumps, Reach and Rake, Arm Swings

Water Walking

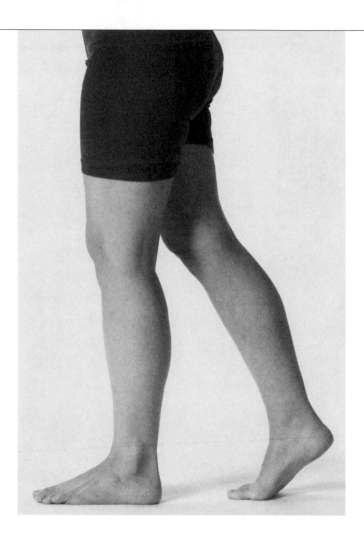

Anyone can do this exercise; it's the most basic water exercise and is easily tolerated. If you do no other exercise but water walking, you are doing something beneficial to your health and wellness. Simply walk the perimeter of the shallow end of the pool using a variety of upper body movements. Start with small steps and gradually increase your stride.

Water Jog

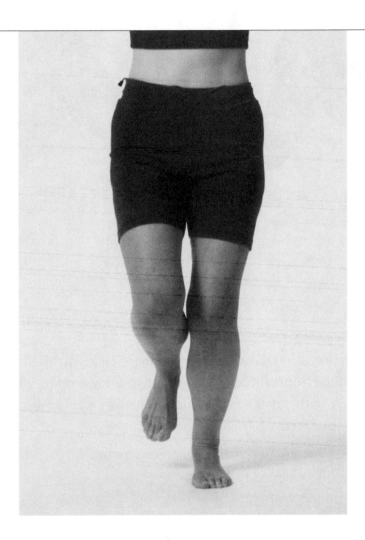

This exercise is a step up from the Prance because the movement is slightly larger and faster. It's important that you bring down your heel with each foot strike and try not to stay up on your toes.

Start jogging in place and progress to jogging around the shallow end of the pool. You can incorporate a variety of upper body exercises with the Water Jog.

Scissors

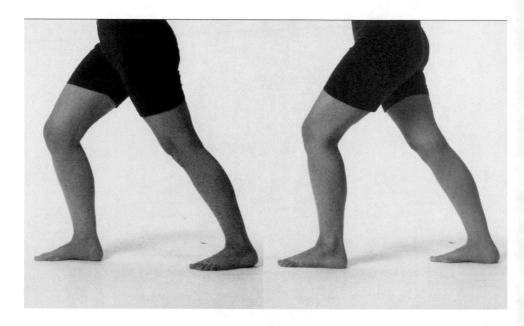

This exercise is like cross-country skiing: Stack your body weight evenly on the front and back leg. Scissor your legs and feet front and back. Start with small scissors and gradually increase the distance between your feet.

Upper body: Pumps, Reach and Rake, Arm Swings

Knee Hops

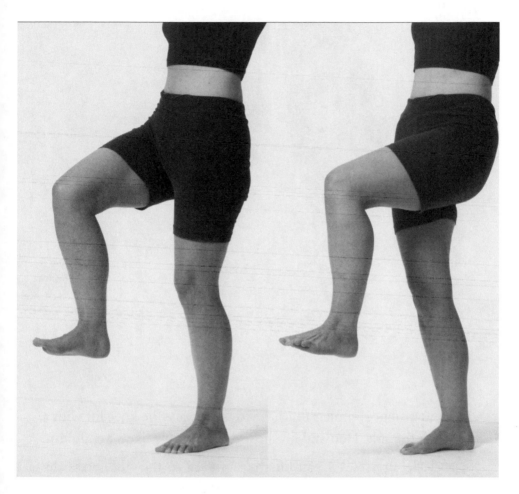

Lift your right knee. Bend your left knee slightly, press off of the pool bottom and hop onto the right leg. Lift your left knee as you hop onto the right foot. The water's buoyancy helps with the hopping action. Keep the knee lift low in the beginning and then, as you feel comfortable, increase the height of the knee lift.

Upper body: Pumps, Arm Swings

Pendulum Swings

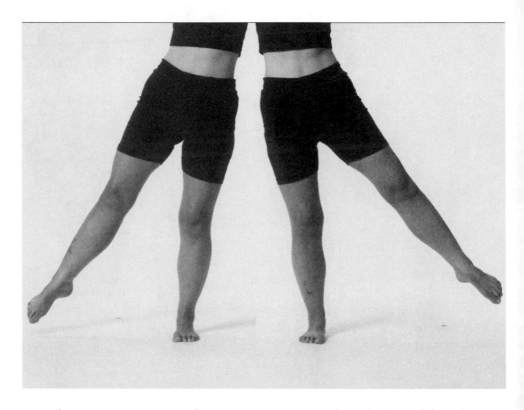

This movement is similar to Knee Hops. Replace the knee lift with a leg lift to the side. Hop and lift the legs side to side like a pendulum.

Upper body: Presses. As you lift the right leg to the side, press the arms down. As you press the left leg to the side, return the arms to the starting position.

Hand position: Windshield Wipers. Your arms should travel in the same direction as the lifted leg.

Jumping Jacks

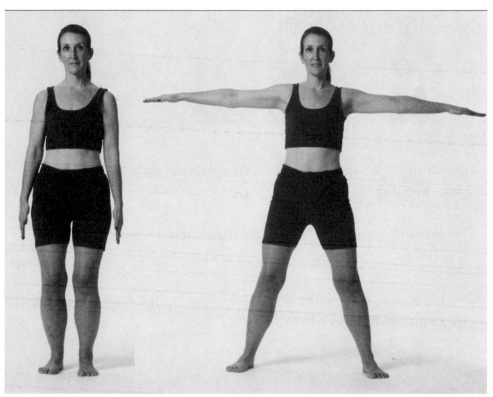

Even if you have never been able to do Jumping Jacks on land, you should be able to do them in water. Begin with your feet together. Jump your feet apart. Jump them together again, and repeat. Your heels should come in contact with the bottom with each jump.

Upper body: Side Lifts, Figure 8s (your arm movement should correspond with your leg movement. When your feet are together your arms should be crossed or close to the body; when your feet are apart, your arms should be open or out to the sides.)

Water Exercise Cool Downs and Stretches

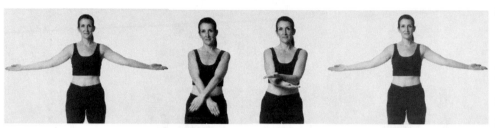

Figure 8s

Once you're finished with your water exercise workout, you'll move into a cool-down and then a stretch.

Stand with your feet a little wider than shoulder width. Slowly do Figures 8s.

Walk to the side of the pool and perform the cool-down and stretching exercises on the following pages.

Cool-Down Exercises

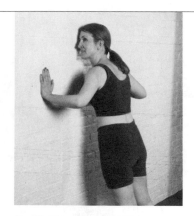

Push-Ups, page 178

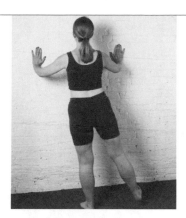

Leg Lifts, page 179

Stretches

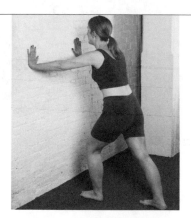

Hamstring Stretch, page 180

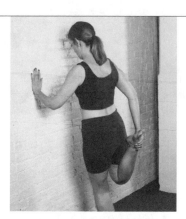

Quadriceps Stretch, page 181

Push-Ups

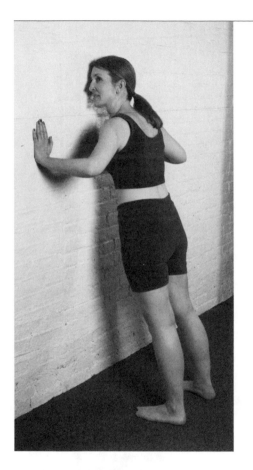 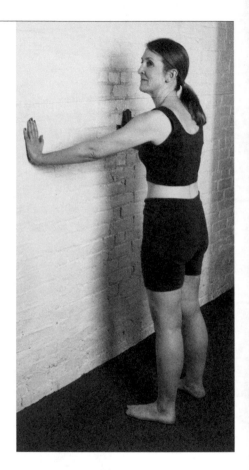

① Face the side of the pool and place both hands on the edge.

② Bend and straighten your elbows slowly and with good control of the movement.

③ Perform 8 to 12 times.

Leg Lifts

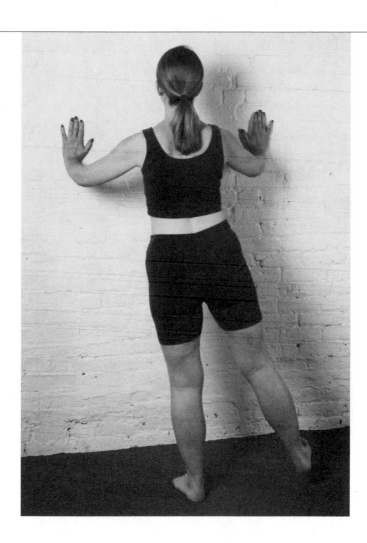

❶ Hold the side of the pool with both hands.

❷ Lift and lower the right leg to the side 8 to 12 times. Repeat with your left leg.

Hamstring Stretch

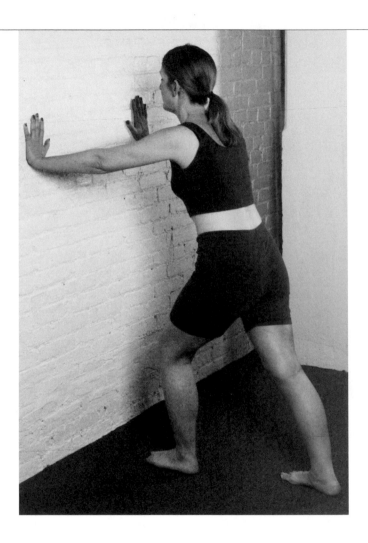

① Hold on to the side of the pool and place one leg in front of the other. Your back leg should be straight and your front knee should be slightly bent.

② Keeping your back heel in contact with the floor, lean forward slightly, until you feel slight tension in your hamstring.

③ Hold the stretch for 20 seconds. Repeat on the opposite leg.

Quadriceps Stretch

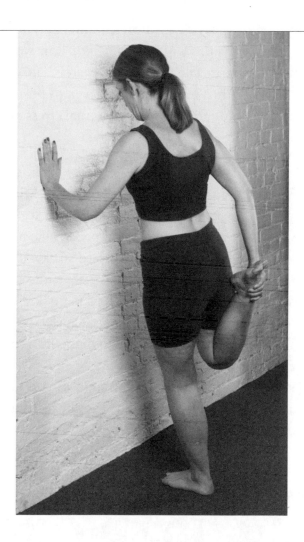

1. Stand a foot or less from the side of the pool.

2. Grasp your right foot with your right hand. Keep your shoulders down and squared-off to the front. You should feel this stretch along the front of your thigh and across your chest and shoulders.

3. Hold for 20 seconds.

Cycling for Cardiovascular Training

Stationary cycling can provide cardiorespiratory conditioning without placing stress on your joints. Since it is a non-weight bearing exercise, cycling is an excellent form of exercise for people with arthritis in their hips. It is important, however, to position yourself correctly on the bike to minimize any potential stress points.

Adjusting Your Stationary Cycle

Seat height. Stand next to the seat of your bike. Adjust the seat height so it is at hip level. Next, sit on the seat, place your feet on the pedals and take a few test revolutions. As you pedal, take notice of your knee when it's straightened on the downward stroke. If your knee is just *slightly* bent, approximately 5 degrees, than the seat height is correct. If your knee is excessively bent, or if the knee lifts higher than hip level, the seat is too low. If the knee locks out or you have to strain to reach the pedals, the seat is too high. Both situations can place a strain on the knee.

    Hand placement. Keep your wrists straight as you grip the handlebars. Your hand, wrist, and forearm should form a line. Don't bend, or break, at the wrist. Keep your grip loose.

Improper Hand Grip

Proper Hand Grip

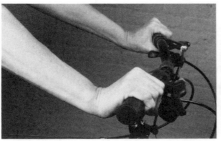
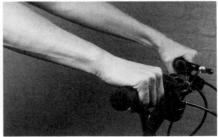

Your elbows should be slightly bent, and your shoulders down and relaxed. Keep your body upright. Don't lean forward and place all your upper body weight onto your arms and hands because this can place stress on the shoulder, elbow, and wrist joints.

Get Ready to Cycle

Pedaling at a light to medium resistance is recommended for people with arthritis. In the workouts in Part III, I don't give specific resistance settings. Rather, I would like you to rely on how the exercise feels. Your best guide is to work at a comfortable pace and resistance below the pain threshold. Pedal with no resistance for the first 5 minutes to warm up. Increase the resistance gradually, until it feels somewhat hard.

Tips to Remember

It's advisable to balance physical activity with periods of rest. You need to pay attention to your body. During periods when symptoms are at their worst, strenuous activities that stress the joints should be avoided.

• Treat yourself to a massage. A massage can help relieve pain and stress. Look for a licensed massage therapist who may have special training or experience working with arthritic clients.

• Hot and cold therapy is another treatment that may help you find relief from your symptoms. Cold therapy involves applying ice to the affected joint for 20 minutes and then removing it for 20 minutes. Continue applying and removing the ice until pain subsides. Heat application for relief of joint stiffness can take the form of a hot shower or bath, hot paraffin (wax) therapy, or warm towels draped over the affected area. Be careful to test the temperature before applying anything hot to your skin.

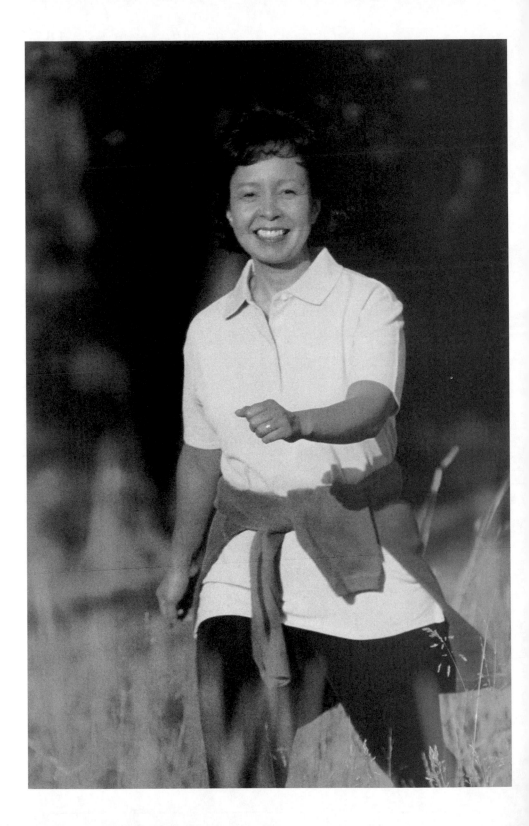

Part III: The Workouts

The Walking Program

The rate at which your walking program progresses will depend on your level of fitness. If you get tired, slow down, and *never* walk in pain.

The following table is a beginner's walking program. Keep in mind that the progression of walking varies from one person to another. Note: If at anytime during exercise you feel dizzy, faint, or experience chest pain, stop immediately and seek the advice of your doctor.

Week	Distance (miles)	Duration (minutes)	Frequency (times per week)
1	.25 to .50	10 to 12	2 to 3
2	.25 to .50	10 to 12	2 to 3
3	.50	12 to 15	2 to 3
4	.50	12 to 15	2 to 3
5	.50 to .75	17 to 20	3
6	.50 to .75	17 to 20	3
7	.75 to 1	20 to 25	3 to 4
8	.75 to 1	20 to 25	3 to 4
9	1 to 1.25	25 to 28	3 to 4
10	1 to 1.25	25 to 28	3 to 4
11	1.25 to 1.50	30 to 34	4
12	1.25 to 1.50	30 to 34	4
13	1.50 to 1.75	35 to 38	4
14	1.50 to 1.75	35 to 38	4
15+	2+	40	4 to 5

The Strength-Training Program

It is difficult to prescribe an exact strength-training program since it depends upon the extent of your arthritis and your tolerance to the exercises. However, I do provide general guidelines and suggest you adjust the program according to your individual needs. Here are some basic guidelines.

+ Strength-training exercises start on page 124.

+ Perform strengthening exercises 2 to 3 times per week.

+ Allow 1 day of rest between strengthening workouts.

Weeks 1 and 2

+ Perform the strengthening exercises (and cardiovascular training) on **Monday** and **Wednesday**.

+ For every exercise, hold each contraction for 3 seconds and repeat the exercise 5 times.

+ When you're able to complete Weeks 1 and 2, progress to Weeks 3 and 4.

Weeks 3 and 4

+ Perform all of the the strengthening exercises on **Monday, Wednesday, and Friday,** in addition to your cardiovascular training.

+ Another approach is to perform the lower body exercises—Seated Cross-Legged Press, Seated Inner Thigh Squeeze, Seated Chest Press, Pelvic Tilt, Prone Leg Lift, Side Leg Lifts, Wall Press, Wall Sitting, and Sit to Stand on one day, and the upper body exercises—Seated Airplanes, Prone Arm Lift, Rubber Band

Stretch, and Sponge Squeeze—on the following day. In other words, each day you will be doing a little aerobic work and some strength training. Performing upper body exercises and lower body exercises on alternating days allows you to rest one body area while working another.

+ Hold each contraction 5 seconds and perform each isometric contraction 8 times.

+ For Sit to Stand, Rubber Band Stretch, and Sponge Squeeze, begin with 5 to 8 repetitions and gradually increase to 12 repetitions.

+ For exercises that suggest the option of using light weights, start with 1- to 2-pound weights and then, if you're able, increase to 4 pounds *after* week 4.

+ If, after several weeks, 4 pounds begins to feel easy, increase to 5 pounds. Progress in this manner through subsequent weeks.

+ The bottom line is to listen to your body and modify the program as needed. The old gym mantra, "No pain, no gain" does not apply to arthritis and exercise.

The Water Exercise Program

There are two ways to approach designing a water program. You can either keep track of the duration of your workout or you can count the number of times you perform each exercise. As you become stronger, increase either the duration of your workout or the number of times you execute the exercise.

To get the benefit of an aerobic water exercise program, try to keep moving for at least 15 minutes. If you get tired, perform only the lower body exercises or only the upper body exercises.

Here's a sample water exercise program that progresses in intensity:

Warm-Up

Warm up for 6 minutes at a slow pace. During the warm-up, perform all arm movements near the surface of the water.

Prance for 2 to 3 minutes: Arm Pumps with Slicers 10 times, Donut 10 times.

Water Walk 2 to 3 minutes: Reach and Rake with Cups 10 times; Arm Swings with Slicers 10 times, with Donuts 10 times.

Aerobics

15 to 20 minutes at a slow to moderate pace.

Water Jog for 2 to 3 minutes. For the upper body movements, do the Arm Pumps with Donuts 10 to 20 times.
Variation 1: Pedal the arms in a circular pattern 10 to 20 times.
Variation 2: Mini-Presses—shorten the range of the motion, but try to increase the speed. 10 to 20 times.

Scissors for 2 to 3 minutes. For the upper body movements:
Arm Pumps with Slicers: 10 to 20 times
Arm Pumps with Donuts: 10 to 20 times
Reach and Rake with Cups: 10 to 20 times
Arm Swings with Slicers: 10 to 20 times
Arm Swings with Donuts: 10 to 20 times

Knee Hops for 2 to 3 minutes. For the upper body movements:
Arm Pumps with Slicers: 10 to 20 times
Arm Pumps with Donuts: 10 to 20 times

Arm Swings with Slicers: 10 to 20 times
Arm Swings with Donuts: 10 to 20 times

Pendulum Swings for 2 to 3 minutes. For the upper body movements:
Presses with Flat Paddles: 10 to 20 times
Windshield Wipers with Slicers: 10 to 20 times

Jumping Jacks for 2 to 3 minutes. For the upper body movements:
Side Raises with Slicers: 10 to 20 times
Side Raises with Flat Paddles: 10 to 20 times
Figure Eights: 10 to 20 times

Cool Down

Cool-down at a slow pace, performing the exercises on pages 176 to 181:

Figure 8s
Push-Ups
Leg Lifts
Hamstring Stretch
Quadriceps Stretch

The Cycling Program

The following is a sample cycling program for you to follow. Overall, your goal is to maintain a slow to moderate pedaling pace for a total of 15 to 20 minutes.

Weeks 1 and 2

	Duration	Resistance	Pedal Rate
Warm-Up	5 minutes	0	Slow
Work Out	15 minutes	Light	Slow
Cooldown	3 minutes	0	Slow

Weeks 3 and 4

	Duration	Resistance	Pedal Rate
Warm-Up	5 minutes	0	Slow
Workout	17 minutes	Light	Slow
Cooldown	3 minutes	0	Slow

Weeks 4 and 5

	Duration	Resistance	Pedal Rate
Warm-Up	5 minutes	0	Slow
Workout	20 minutes	Light–medium	Slow
Cooldown	3 minutes	0	Slow

Weeks 6 and 7

	Duration	Resistance	Pedal Rate
Warm-Up	5 minutes	0	Slow
Workout	20 minutes	light–medium	Moderate
Cooldown	3 minutes	0	Slow

Adjust the time, resistance, and pedaling pace according to how you feel. Listen to your body.

Once you have a good understanding of proper form and positioning on the stationary bike and have established a baseline of conditioning, you're ready to add upper body exercises that can be done while you pedal. (Of course, if you're riding a moving bike, you won't be able to add upper body exercises).

Start with the Range of Motion exercises that start on page 80. These can be done during the warm-up. Some of the Strength-Training exercises that start on page 124 can be performed on the bike as you pedal. Do the exercises one arm at a time, maintaining balance and support with the other arm.

References

Boulware D.W., Byrd S.L., "Optimizing Exercise Programs for Arthritis Patients," (1993). *Physicians and Sports Medicine.*

Samples, P., "Exercises Encouraged for People with Arthritis." (1990). *Physician and Sports Medicine.*

Neiman, D., "Exercise Soothes Arthritis Joint Effects." (2000). *American College of Sports Medicine, Health Fitness Journal*

Smeltzer, S. and Bare, B. (2000). Brunner & Suddarth's Medical Surgical Nursing. (9th ed.) Philadelphia: Lippincott.

Glossary

analgesic A medication or treatment that relieves pain.

arthritis Literally means joint inflammation, but is often used to indicate a group of more than 100 rheumatic diseases. These diseases affect not only the joints but also other connective tissues of the body, including important supporting structures such as muscles, tendons, and ligaments, as well as the protective covering of internal organs.

autoimmune disease One in which the immune system destroys or attacks the patient's own body tissue.

cartilage A tough, resilient tissue that covers and cushions the ends of the bones and absorbs shock.

chronic disease An illness that lasts for a long time.

collagen The main structural protein of skin, tendon, bone cartilage, and connective tissues.

connective tissue The supporting framework of the body and its internal organs.

fibromyalgia Sometimes called fibrositis, a chronic disorder that causes pain and stiffness throughout the tissues that support and move the bones and joints. Pain and localized tender points occur in the muscles, particularly those that support the neck, spine, shoulders, and hips. The disorder includes widespread pain, fatigue, and sleep disturbances.

fibrous capsule A tough wrapping of tendons and ligaments that surrounds the joint.

flare A period in which disease symptoms reappear or become worse.

genetic marker A specific tissue type or gene, similar to a blood type, that is passed on from parents to their children. Some genetic markers are linked to certain rheumatic diseases.

immune response The reaction of the immune system against foreign substances. When this reaction occurs against substances or tissues within the body, it is called an autoimmune reaction.

immune system A complex system that normally protects the body from infections. It combines groups of cells, the chemicals that control them, and the chemicals they release.

inflammation A characteristic reaction of tissues to injury or disease. It is marked by four signs: swelling, redness, heat, and pain.

joint A junction where two bones meet. Most joints are composed of cartilage, joint space, fibrous capsule, synovium, and ligaments.

joint space The volume enclosed within the fibrous capsule and synovium.

ligaments Bands of cordlike tissue that connect bone to bone.

muscle A structure composed of bundles of specialized cells that, when stimulated by nerve impulses, contract and produce movement.

myopathies Inflammatory and noninflammatory diseases of muscle.

myositis Inflammation of a muscle.

nonsteroidal anti-inflammatory drugs (NSAIDs) A group of drugs, such as aspirin and aspirin-like drugs, used to reduce inflammation that causes joint pain, stiffness, and swelling.

Raynaud's phenomenon A circulatory condition associated with spasms in the blood vessels of the fingers and toes causing them to change color. After exposure to cold, these areas turn white, then blue, and finally red.

remission A period during which symptoms of disease are reduced (partial remission) or disappear (complete remission).

sicca syndrome A condition manifested by dry eyes and dry mouth.

sleep disorder One in which a person has difficulty achieving restful, restorative sleep. In addition to other symptoms, patients with fibromyalgia usually have a sleep disorder.

synovium A tissue that surrounds and protects the joints. It produces synovial fluid that nourishes and lubricates the joints.

tender points Specific locations on the body that are painful, especially when pressed.

tendons Fibrous cords that connect muscle to bone.

vasculitis Inflammation in the blood vessels. It may occur throughout the body.

Resources

ORGANIZATIONS

National Institute of Arthritis and Musculoskeletal and Skin Diseases Information Clearinghouse
National Institutes of Health

1 AMS Circle
Bethesda, MD 20892-3675
Phone: 301-495-4484 or 877-22-NIAMS (226-4267) (free of charge)
TTY: 301-565-2966
Fax: 301-718-6366
http://www.niams.nih.gov/

The clearinghouse provides information about various forms of arthritis and rheumatic disease and bone, muscle, and skin diseases. It distributes patient and professional education materials and refers people to other sources of information. Additional information and updates can also be found on the NIAMS Web site.

American Academy of Orthopaedic Surgeons

P.O. Box 2058
Des Plaines, IL 60017
Phone: 800-824-BONE (2663) (free of charge)
www.aaos.org

The academy provides education and practice management services for orthopaedic surgeons and allied health professionals. It also serves as an advocate for improved patient care and informs the public about the science of orthopaedics. The orthopaedist's scope of practice includes disorders of the body's bones, joints, ligaments, muscles, and tendons. For a single copy of an AAOS brochure, send a self-addressed stamped envelope to the address above or visit the AAOS Web site.

American College of Rheumatology
1800 Century Place, Suite 250
Atlanta, GA 30345
Phone: 404-633-3777
Fax: 404-633-1870
www.rheumatology.org

This association provides referrals to doctors and health professionals
who work on arthritis, rheumatic diseases, and related conditions. The
association also provides educational materials and guidelines.

American Physical Therapy Association
1111 North Fairfax Street
Alexandria, VA 22314-1488
Phone: 703-684-2782 or 800-999-2782, ext. 3395 (free of charge)
www.apta.org

The association is a national professional organization representing physical therapists, allied personnel, and students. Its objectives are to improve
research, public understanding, and education in the physical therapies.

The Aquatic Exercise Association
P.O. Box 1609
Nokomis, FL 34274
941-486-8600
www.aeawave.com

Arthritis Foundation
1330 West Peachtree Street
Atlanta, GA 30309
Phone: 404-872-7100 or 800-283-7800 (free of charge) or
call your local chapter (listed in the telephone directory)
www.arthritis.org

This is the major voluntary organization devoted to arthritis. The foundation publishes a free pamphlet on exercise and arthritis and a monthly
magazine for members that provides up-to-date information on all
forms of arthritis. Local chapters organize exercise programs for people
who have arthritis, including People with Arthritis Can Exercise (PACE)

and an aquatic exercise program held in swimming pools. The foundation also can provide physician and clinic referrals.

Fibromyalgia Network
P.O. Box 31750
Tucson, AZ 85751-1750
800/853-2929
Contact: Ms. Kristin Thorson

Fibromyalgia Partnership (formerly Fibromyalgia Association of Greater Washington)
P.O. Box 160
Linden, VA 22642-0160
(toll free) 866/725-4404
Fax: 866-666-2727
www.fmpartnership.org

PACE Catalog Center
Arthritis Foundation
P.O. Box 9020
Pittsfield, MA 01202-9945
Phone: 800-PACE-236 (722-3236) (free of charge)

This center sells PACE exercise videotapes at two levels, basic and advanced. Each videotape is approximately 30 minutes long and includes a warm-up section, a gentle or moderate exercise routine, and a rhythmic movement sequence to help improve endurance. The videotapes are available for $19.50 per tape, plus shipping charges.

Lupus Foundation of America, Inc. (LFA)
2000 L Street, N.W., Suite 710
Washington, DC 20036
Phone: 202-349-1155
Toll Free: (800)558-0121
Fax: 202-349-1156
E-mail: lupusinfo@lupus.org
www.lupus.org

This is the main voluntary organization devoted to lupus. It also provides information on arthritis and exercise.

SLE Foundation
149 Madison Avenue, Suite 205
New York, NY 10016
Phone: 212-685-4118
www.lupusny.org

This foundation supports and encourages medical research to find the cause and cure of lupus and improve its diagnosis and treatment. It also provides information on arthritis and exercise.

National Fibromyalgia Partnership, Inc.
140 Zinn Way
Linden, VA 22642-5609
Phone: 866-725-4404 (free of charge)
Fax: 540-622-2998
E-mail: mail@fmpartnership.org
www.fmpartnership.org

This organization devoted to fibromyalgia provides information on arthritis and exercise.

Spondylitis Association of America (SAA)
P.O. Box 5872
Sherman Oaks, CA 91413
Phone: 818-981-1616 or 800-777-8189 (free of charge)
www.spondylitis.org

This nonprofit, voluntary organization helps people who have ankylosing spondylitis and related conditions. SAA sells books, posters, videotapes, and audiotapes about exercises for people who have arthritis of the spine.

FITNESS GEAR

Hydro-Fit Aquatic Fitness Gear
1328 West 2nd Ave.
Eugene, OR 97402
1-800-346-7295
http://www.hydrofit.com

Developer and manufacturer of aquatic health and fitness products. The Company's unique product line provides enhanced buoyancy and increased resistance for water aerobics, water exercise, and aquatic therapy.

Speedo
www.speedo.com
Swimwear, including aquatic sports shoes.

Splash International
888-775-2744
http://splashinternational.com
Swimwear, accessories, and exercise equipment.

VIDEOS

Move It or Lose It: Arthritis Water Fitness
Fibromyalgia Waterwork with Mary Essert

Essert Associates
3635 Irby Drive
Conway, AR 72034
E-mail: messert@mindspring.com.